Table of Contents

C000083649

Skeletal System

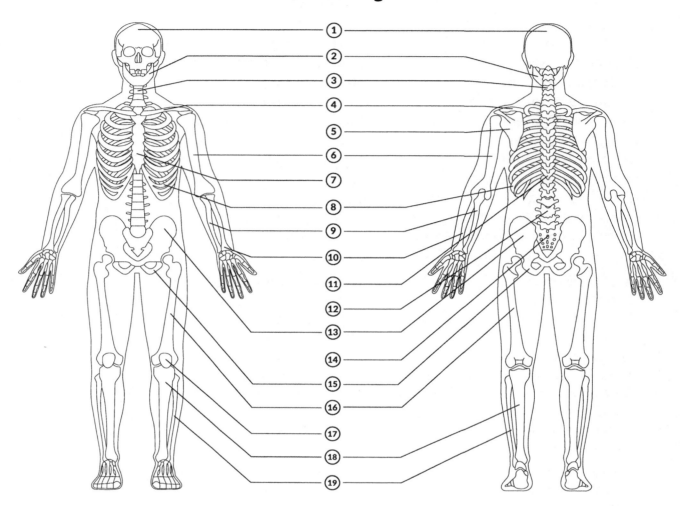

- - Answer - -

(1). Skull

(2). Mandible

(3). Cervical vertebrae

(4). Clavicle

(5). Scapula

(6). Humerus

(7). Sternum

(8). Rib

(9). Ulna

(10). Radius

(11). Thoracic vertebrae

(12). Lumbar vertebrae

(13). Ilium

(14). Sacrum

(15). Ischium

(16). Femur

(17). Patella

(18). Tibia

(19). Fibula

Muscular System

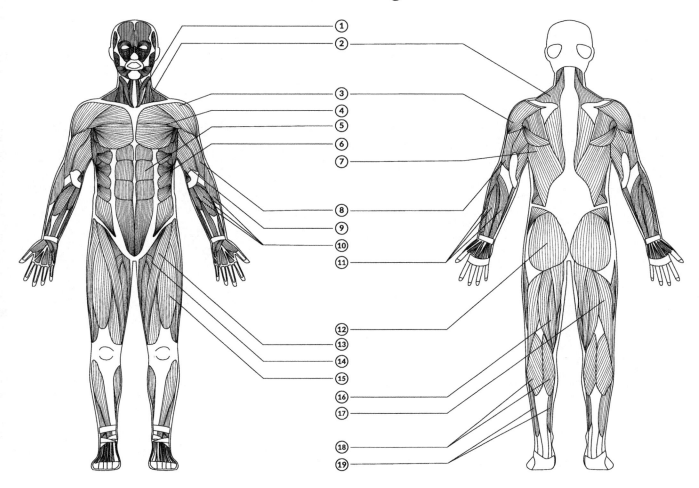

- - Answer - -

(1). Sternocleidomastoid

(2). Trapezius

(3). Deltoid

(4). Pectoralis Major

(5). Rectus Abdominis

(6). External Oblique

(7). Latissimus Dorsi

(8). Triceps Brachii

(9). Biceps Brachii

(10). Finger Flexors

(11). Finger Extensors

(12). Gluteus Maximus

(13). Sartorius

(14). Adductor Longus

(15). Rectus Femoris

(16). Semimembranosus

(17). Biceps Femoris

(18). Gastrocnemius

(19). Soleus

Immune System

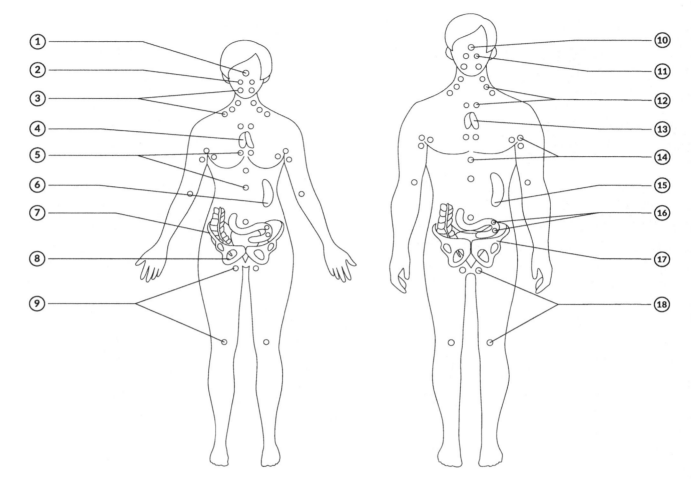

- - Answer - -

(1). Tonsils

(2). Adenoids

(3). Lymph Nodes

(4). Thymus

(5). Lymph Nodes

(6). Spleen

(7). Bone Marrow

(8). Appendix

(9). Lymph Nodes

(10). Tonsils

(11). Adenoids

(12). Lymph Nodes

(13). Thymus

(14). Lymph Nodes

(15). Spleen

(16). Peyer's Patches

(17). Bone Marrow

(18). Lymph Nodes

Nervous System

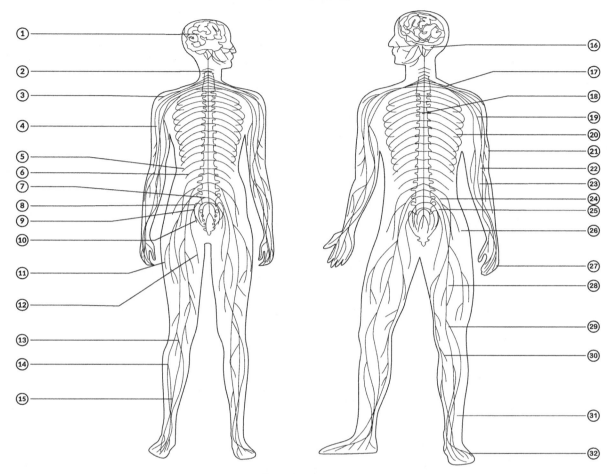

- - Answer - -

(1). Cerebral Hemisphere

(2). Cervical Plexus

(3). Suprascapular Nerve

(4). Axillary Nerve

(5). Iliac-Hypogastric Nerve

(6). Iliac Inguinal Nerve

(7). Ponytail

(8). Femoral Nerve

(9). Gluteal Nerves

(10). Coccygeal Nerves

(11). Posterior Cutaneous
Nerve of The Thigh

(12). Obstructive Nerve

(13). Calf Nerve

(14). Superficial Peroneal Nerve

(15). Deep Fibular Nerve

(16). Cerebellum

(17). Brachial Plexus

(18). Spinal Cord

(19). Musculocutaneous Nerve

(20). Intercostal Nerve

(21). Radial Nerve

(22). Ulnar Nerve

(23). Median Nerve

(24). Lumbar Plexus

(25). Sacral Plexus

(26). Lateral Cutaneous
Nerve of The Thigh

(27). Finger Nerves

(28). Sciatic Nerve

(29). Common Peroneal Nerve

(30). Saphenous Nerve

(31). Tibial Nerve

(32). Toe Nerves

Endocrine System

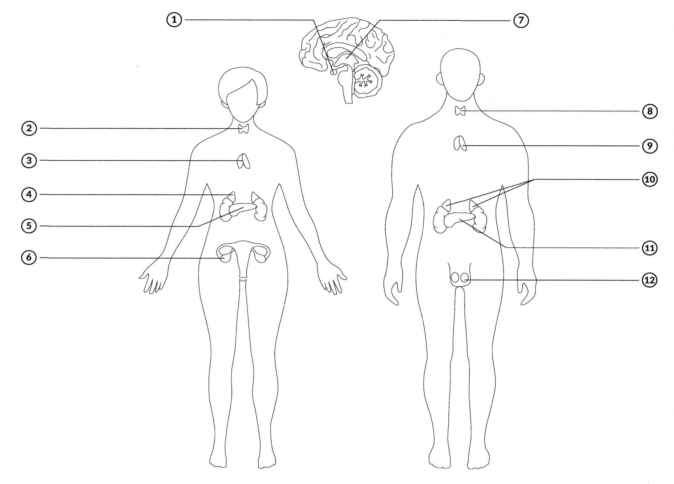

- - Answer - -

(1). Pituitary Gland

(2). Thyroid Gland

(3). Thymus

(4). Adrenal Glands

(5). Pancreas

(6). Ovaries

(7). Hypothalamus

(8). Thyroid Gland

(9). Thymus

(10). Adrenal Glands

(11). Pancreas

(12). Testies

Cardiovascular System

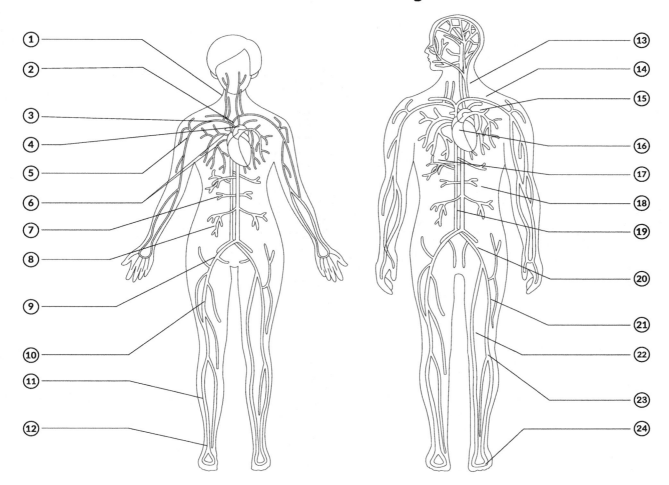

- - Answer - -

(1). Carotid Artery

(2). Brachiocephalic Artery

(3). Subclavian Artery

(4). Aorta

(5). Axillary Artery

(6). Pulmonary Veins

(7). Renal Artery

(8). Mesenteric Artery

(9). External Illiac Artery

(10). Femoral Artery

(11). Posterior Tibial Artery

(12). Anterior Tibial Artery

(13). Jugular Vein

(14). Subclavian Vein

(15). Pulmonary Artery

(16). Heart

(17). Hepatic Veins

(18). Renal Vein

(19). Inferior Vena Cava

(20). Common Iliac Vein

(21). Femoral Vein

(22). Great Saphenous Vein

(23). Popliteal Vein

(24). Dorsal Venous Arch

Lymphatic System

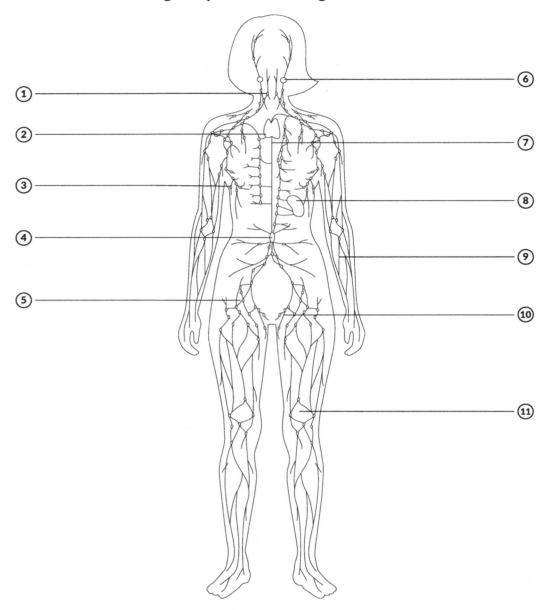

- - Answer - -

(1). Cervical Lymph Nodes

(2). Thymus

(3). Axillary Lymph Nodes

(4). Cisterna Chyli

(5). Pelvic Lymph Nodes

(6). Tonsil

(7). Thoratic Duct

(8). Spleen

(9). Lymphatic Vessels

(10). Inguinal Lymph Nodes

(11). Porliteal Lymph Nodes

Lymphatic System

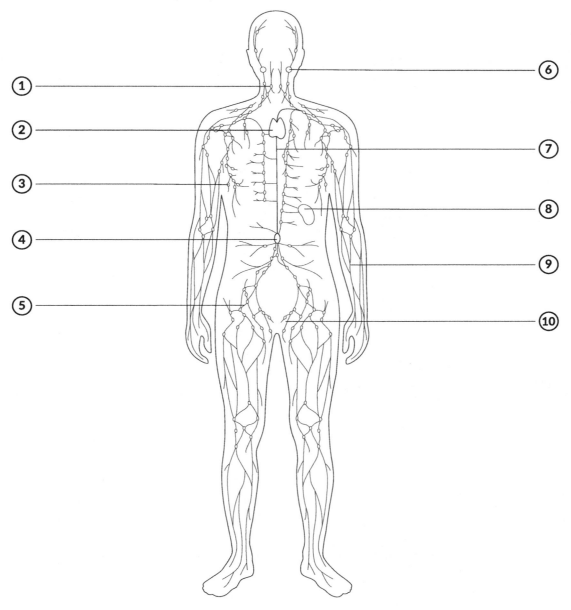

- - Answer - -

(1). **Cervical Lymph Nodes**

(2). **Thymus**

(3). **Axillary Lymph Nodes**

(4). **Cisterna Chyli**

(5). **Pelvic Lymph Nodes**

(6). **Tonsil**

(7). **Thoratic Duct**

(8). **Spleen**

(9). **Lymphatic Vessels**

(10). **Inguinal Lymph Nodes**

Digestive System

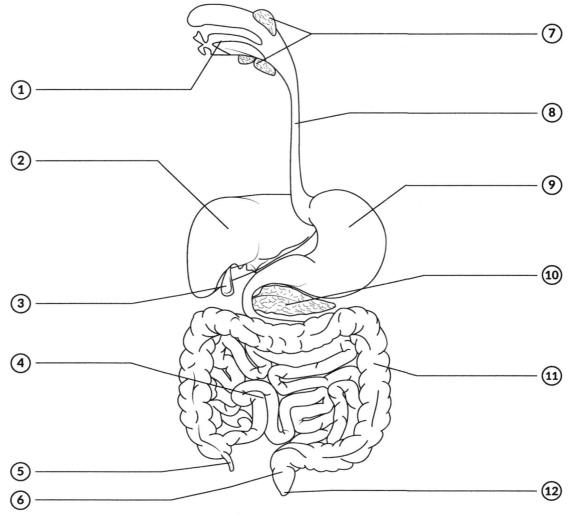

- - Answer - -

(1). Mouth

(2). Liver

(3). Gall Bladder

(4). Small Intestine

(5). Appendix

(6). Rectum

(7). Salivary Glands

(8). Esophagus

(9). Stomach

(10). Pancreas

(11). Large Intestine

(12). Anus

Respiratory System

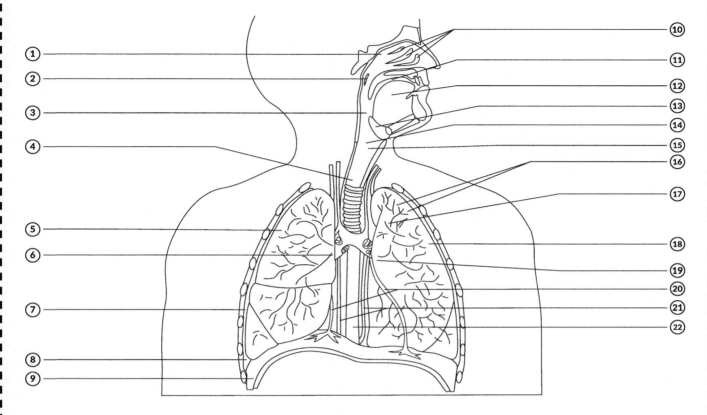

- - Answer - -

(1). Nasal Cavity

(2). Pharyngeal Opening of Pharyngotympanic (Auditory) Tube

(3). Pharynx

(4). Trachea

(5). Right Lung

(6). Right Bronchus

(7). Parietal Pleura

(8). Pleural Cavity

(9). Diaphragm

(10). Nasal Conchae

(11). Oral Cavity

(12). Tongue

(13). Epiglottis

(14). Vocal Folds

(15). Larynx

(16). Terminal Bronchioles

(17). Bronchioles

(18). Left Lung

(19). Left Bronchus

(20). Phrenic Nerves

(21). Vagus Nerves

(22). Esophagus

Integumentary System

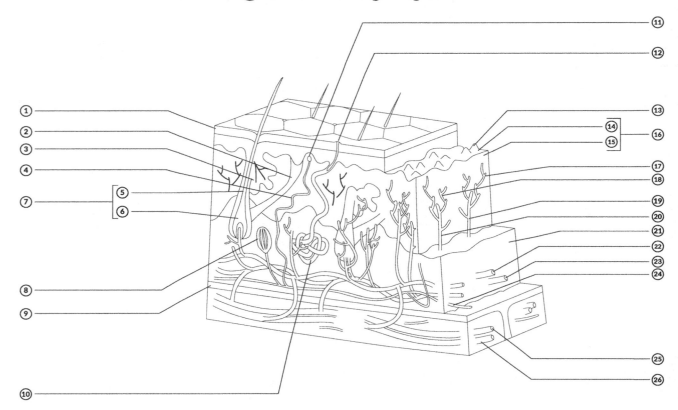

- - Answer - -

(1). Epidermis

(2). Arrector Pili Muscle

(3). Sebaceous Gland

(4). Free Nerve Ending

(5). Hair Shaft

(6). Hair Follicle

(7). Hair

(8). Lamellar Corpuscle

(9). Deep Fascia

(10). Sweat Gland

(11). Tactile Corpuscle

(12). Sweat Pore

(13). Dermal Papillae

(14). Papillary Layer

(15). Reticular Layer

(16). Dermis

(17). Subpapillary Arterial Plexus

(18). Subpapillary Venous Plexus

(19). Deep Dermal Arterial Plexus

(20). Deep Dermal Venous Plexus

(21). Subcutaneous Tissue

(22). Subcutaneous Venous Plexus

(23). Subcutaneous Arterial Plexus

(24). Subcutaneous Neural Plexus

(25). Intramuscular Vein

(26). Intramuscular Artery

Urinary System

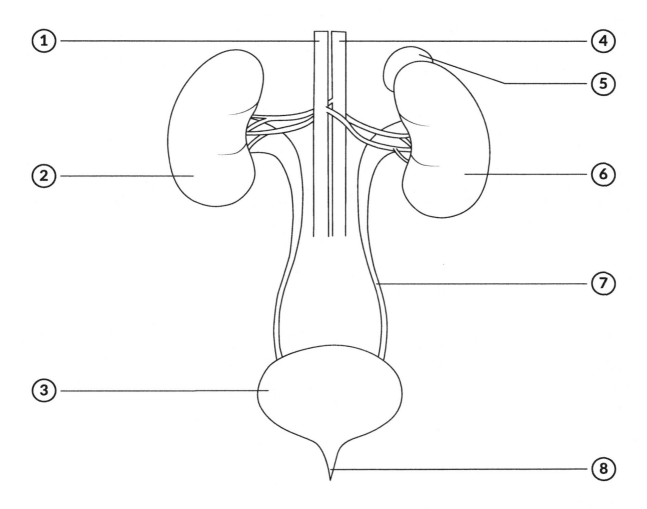

- - Answer - -

(1).Inferior Vena Cava

(2).Right Kidney

(3).Bladder

(4).Descending Aorta

(5).Adrenal Gland

(6).Left Kidney

(7).Ureter

(8).Urethra

Female Reproductive System

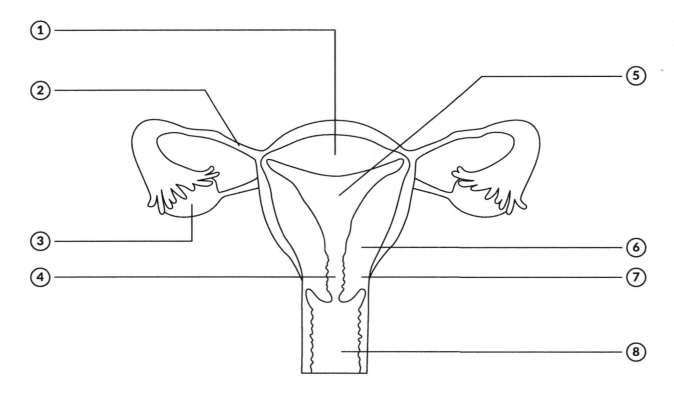

- - Answer - -

(1). Fundus of Uterus

(2). Fallopian Tube

(3). Ovary

(4). Cervical Canal

(5). Uterus

(6). Myometrium

(7). Cervix

(8). Vagina

Male Reproductive System

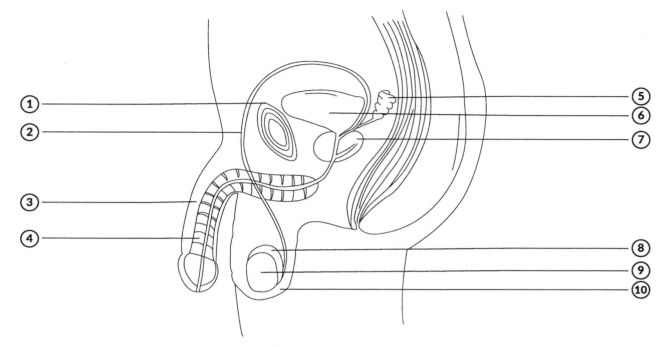

- - Answer - -

(1). Pubic Bone

(2). Ductus Deferens

(3). Penis

(4). Spongy Urethra

(5). Seminal Vesicle

(6). Bladder

(7). Prostate Gland

(8). Epididymis

(9). Testis

(10). Scrotum

Heart and Blood Circulation System

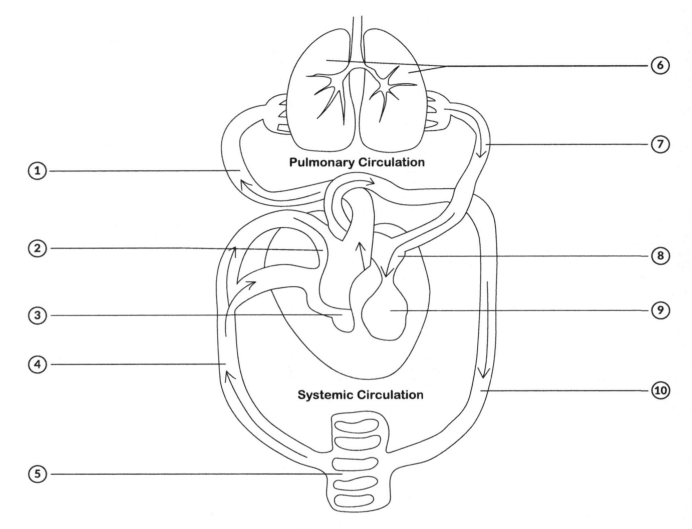

- - Answer - -

(1). Pulmonary Artery

(2). Right Atrium

(3). Right Ventricle

(4). Venae Cavae

(5). Capillaries

(6). Lungs

(7). Pulmonary Artery

(8). Left Atrium

(9). Left Ventricle

(10). Aorta

Internal Organs

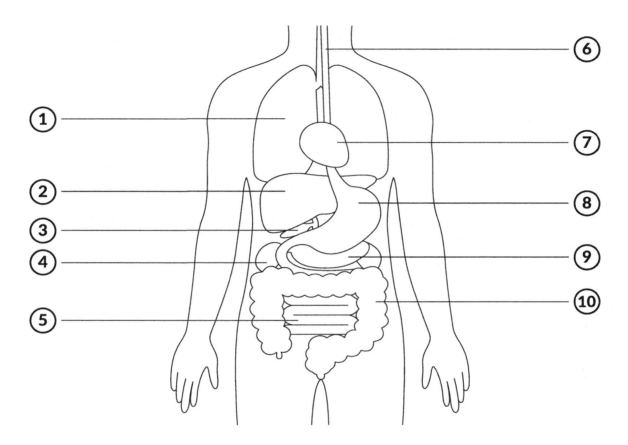

-- Answer --

(1). Lungs

(2). Liver

(3). Gallbladder

(4). Kidney

(5). Small Intestines

(6). Esophagus

(7). Heart

(8). Stomach

(9). Pancreas

(10). Large Intestine

Mouth

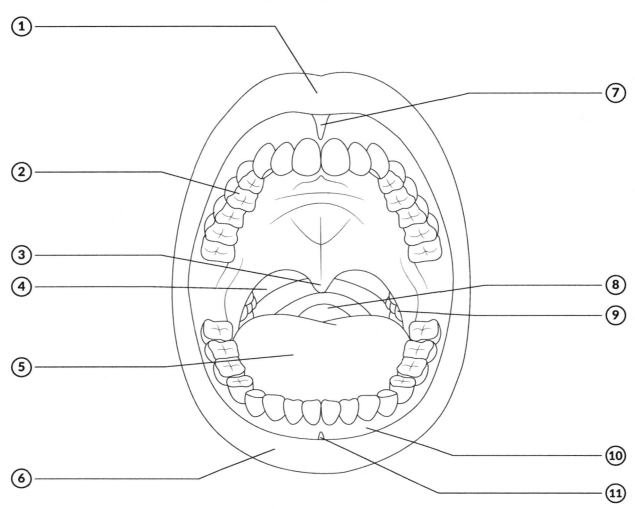

- - Answer - -

(1). Upper Lip

(2). Teeth

(3). Uvula

(4). Pharyngopalatine Arch

(5). Tongue

(6). Lower Lip

(7). Superior Labial Frenulum

(8). Fauces

(9). Palatine Tonsil

(10). Gingivae

(11). Inferior Labial Frenulum

Human Dental Anatomy

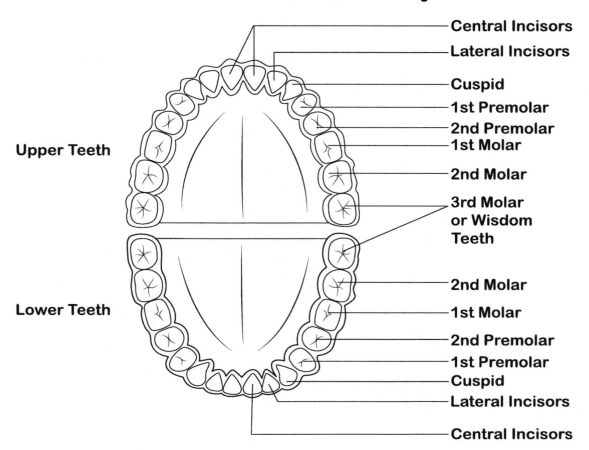

Upper Teeth

Central Incisors
Lateral Incisors
Cuspid
1st Premolar
2nd Premolar
1st Molar
2nd Molar
3rd Molar or Wisdom Teeth

Lower Teeth

2nd Molar
1st Molar
2nd Premolar
1st Premolar
Cuspid
Lateral Incisors
Central Incisors

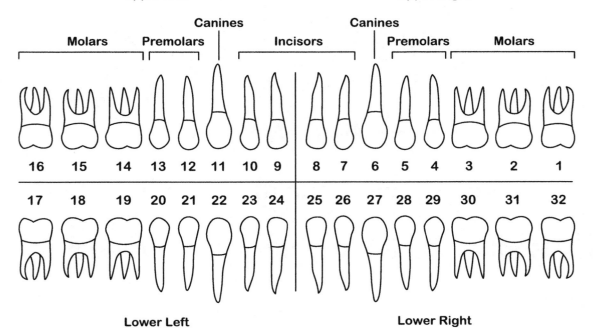

Upper Left   Upper Right

Canines   Canines

Molars   Premolars   Incisors   Premolars   Molars

16 15 14 13 12 11 10 9 8 7 6 5 4 3 2 1

17 18 19 20 21 22 23 24 25 26 27 28 29 30 31 32

Lower Left   Lower Right

Tooth

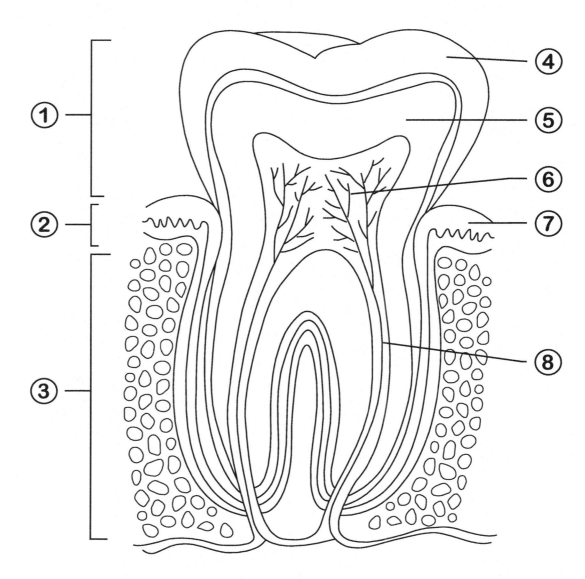

-- Answer --

(1). Crown   (4). Enamel   (7). Gingiva

(2). Neck   (5). Dentin   (8). Root Canal

(3). Root   (6). Pulp Cavity

Eye

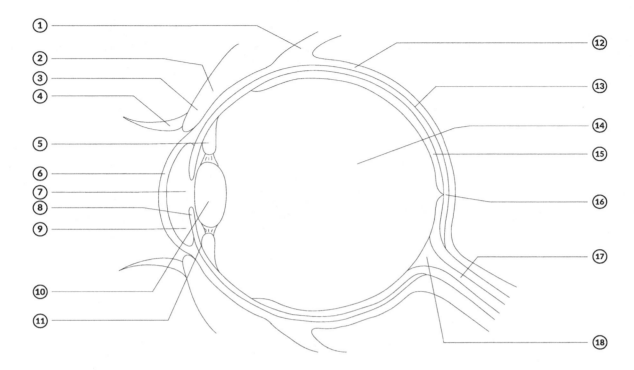

-- Answer --

(1). **Rectus Muscle**

(2). **Conjuctiva**

(3). **Eyelid**

(4). **Eyelash**

(5). **Ciliary Body**

(6). **Cornea**

(7). **Pupil**

(8). **Iris**

(9). **Aqueous Chamber**

(10). **Lense**

(11). **Suspensory Ligament**

(12). **Sclera**

(13). **Choroid**

(14). **Vitreuous Humour**

(15). **Retina**

(16). **Fovea**

(17). **Optic Nerve**

(18). **Blind Spot**

Ear

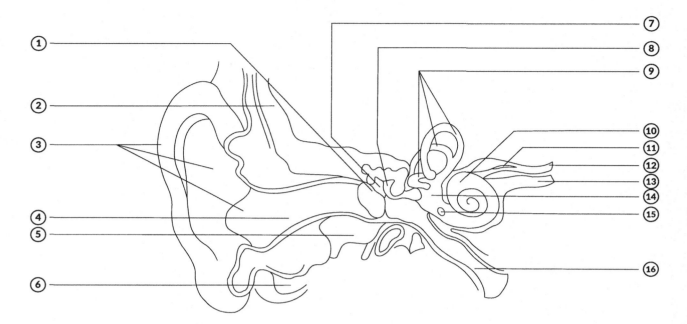

EXTERNAL EAR   MIDDLE EAR   INTERNAL EAR

-- Answer --

(1). Tympanic Membrane

(2). Temporal Bone

(3). Auricle

(4). External Auditory Meatus

(5). Temporal Bone

(6). Mastoid Air Cells

(7). Malleus

(8). Incus

(9). Semicircular Canals

(10). Cochlea

(11). Facial Nerve

(12). Vestibular Nerve

(13). Cochlear Nerve

(14). Vestibule

(15). Round Window

(16). Auditory Tube (Eustachian Tube)

Ear

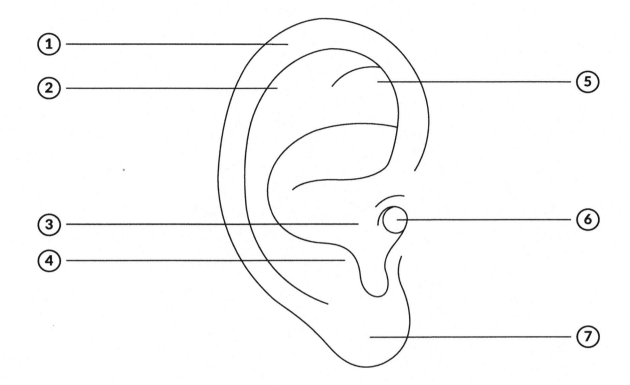

-- Answer --

(1). Helix   (5). Fossa

(2). Scapha   (6). External Auditory Canal

(3). Concha   (7). Lobule

(4). Antitragus

Nose

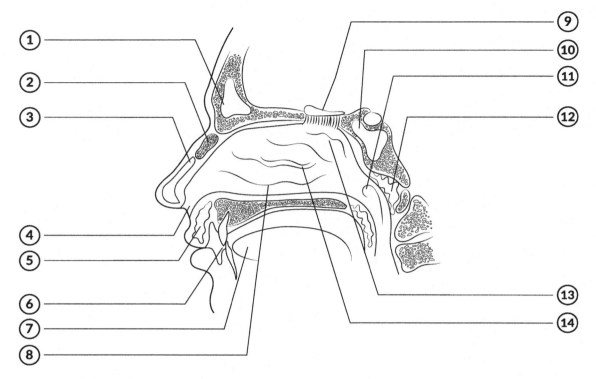

-- Answer --

(1). Frontal Sinus

(2). Nasal Bone

(3). Cartilage

(4). Nasal Cavity

(5). Lip Muscle

(6). Teeth

(7). Tongue

(8). Inferior Nasal Concha

(9). Olfactory Bulb

(10). Sphenoidal Sinus

(11). Nasopharynx

(12). Pharyngeal Tonsil

(13). Nasal Concha

(14). Middle Nasal Concha

Tongue

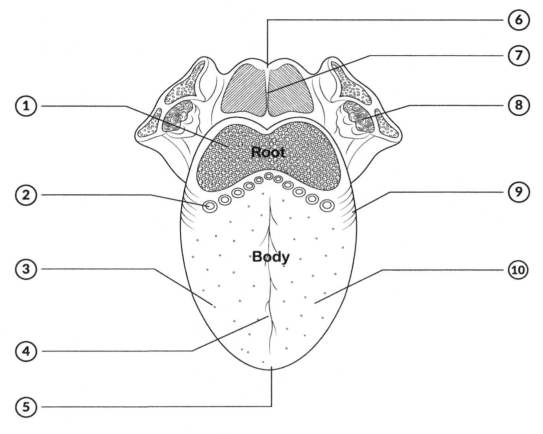

-- Answer --

(1). Lingual tonsil

(2). Vallate papillae

(3). Filiform papillae

(4). Median lingual sulcus

(5). Apex

(6). Epiglottis

(7). Median glosso-epiglottic fold

(8). Palatine tonsil

(9). Foliate papillae

(10). Fungiform papillae

Brain

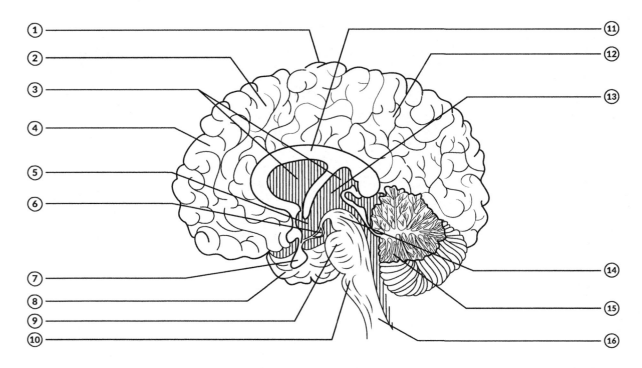

① ② ③ ④ ⑤ ⑥ ⑦ ⑧ ⑨ ⑩ ⑪ ⑫ ⑬ ⑭ ⑮ ⑯

-- Answer --

(1). Cerebral cortex

(2). Cerebrum

(3). Ventricles

(4). Frontal lobe

(5). Hypothalamus

(6). Mammillary body

(7). Pituitary gland

(8). Temporal lobe

(9). Pons

(10). Medulla

(11). Corpus callosum

(12). Parietal lobe

(13). Thalamus

(14). Midbrain

(15). Cerebellum

(16). Brain stem

Heart

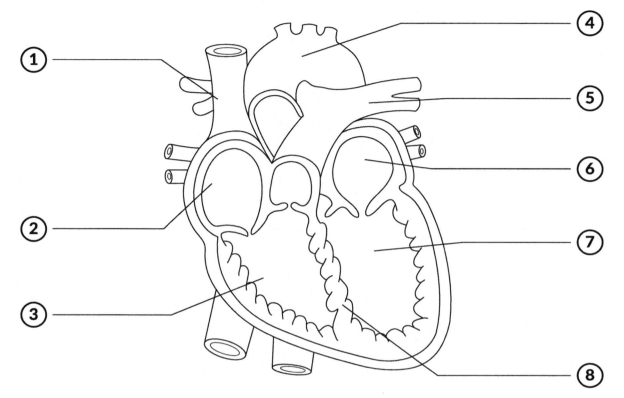

-- Answer --

(1). **Superior Vena Cava**

(2). **Right Atrium**

(3). **Right Ventricle**

(4). **Aorta**

(5). **Pulmonary Artery**

(6). **Left Atrium**

(7). **Left Ventricle**

(8). **Interventricular Septum**

Heart And Lungs

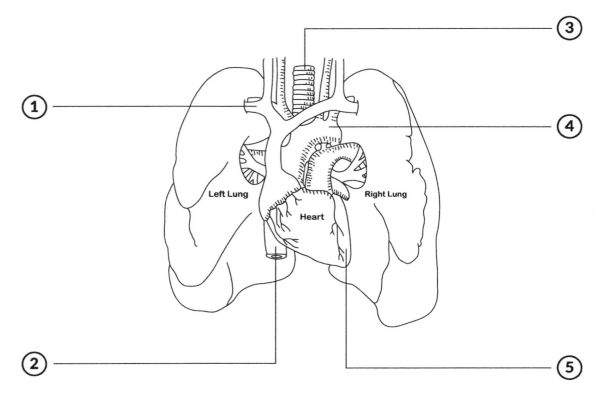

-- Answer --

(1). Superior Vena Cava

(2). Inferior Vena Cava

(3). Trachea

(4). Aorta

(5). Apex of Heart

Liver

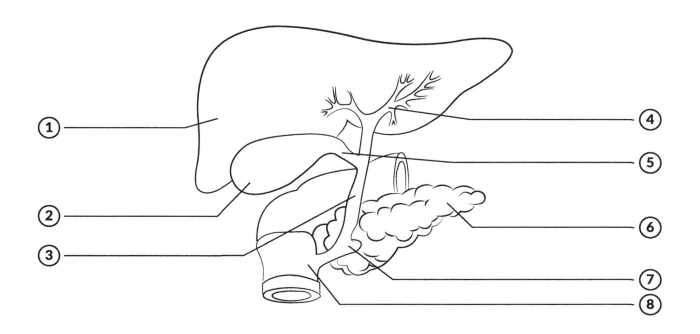

-- Answer --

(1). Liver

(2). Gallbladder

(3). Common bile duct

(4). Hepatic ducts

(5). Cystic duct

(6). Pancreas

(7). Pancreatic duct

(8). Duodenum

Kidney

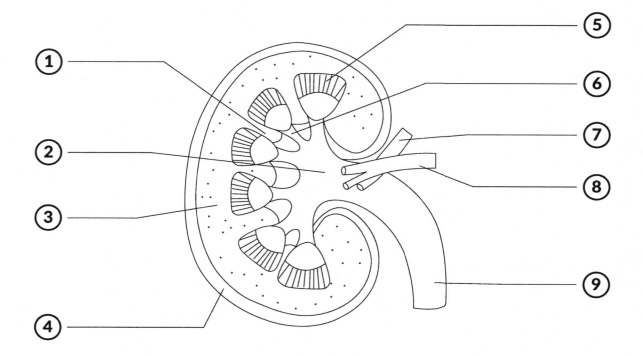

-- Answer --

(1). Renal Column

(2). Renal Pelvis

(3). Cortex

(4). Renal Capsule

(5). Medullary Pyramid

(6). Calyx

(7). Renal Artery

(8). Renal Vein

(9). Ureter

Pancreas

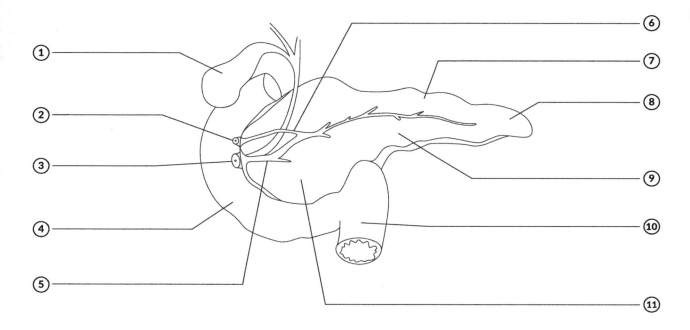

- - Answer - -

(1). **Gallbladder**

(2). **Minor Duodenal Papilla**

(3). **Major Duodenal Papilla**

(4). **Deodenum**

(5). **Main Pancreatic Duct**

(6). **Accessory Pancreatic Duct**

(7). **Pancreas**

(8). **Tail**

(9). **Body**

(10). **Jejunum**

(11). **Head**

Stomach

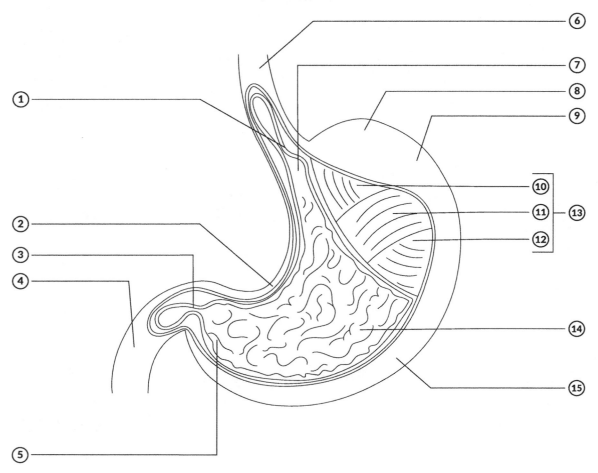

- - Answer - -

(1). Lower esophageal Sphincter

(2). Lesser Curvature

(3). Pyloric Sphincter

(4). Deodenum

(5). Pylorus

(6). Esophagus

(7). Cardia

(8). Fundus

(9). Body of Stomach

(10). Longitudinal Layer

(11). Circular Layer

(12). Oblique Layer

(13). Muscularis externa

(14). Rugae of Stomach

(15). Greater Curvature

Skin

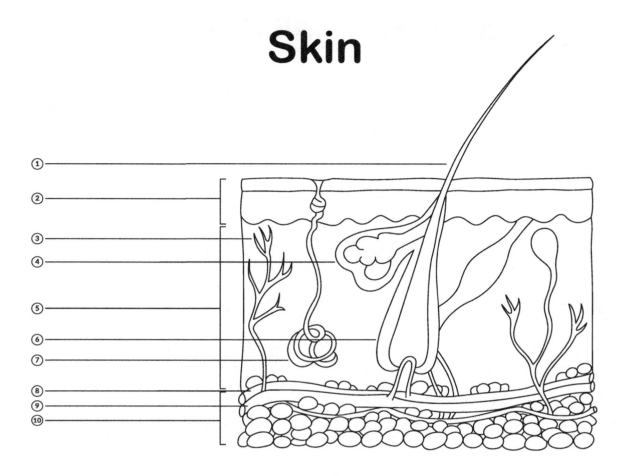

-- Answer --

(1). Hair Shaft

(2). Epidermis

(3). Nerve

(4). Sebaceous Gland

(5). Dermis

(6). Hair Follicle

(7). Sweat Gland

(8). Vein

(9). Artery

(10). Subcutaneous Layer

Large & Small Intestine

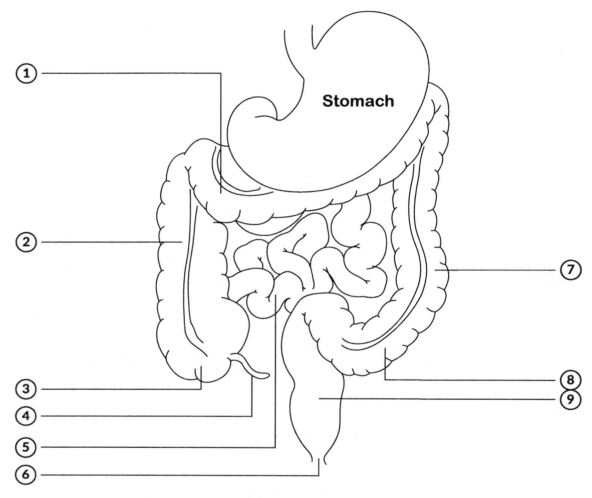

Stomach

-- Answer --

(1). Transverse Colon

(2). Ascending Colon

(3). Cecum

(4). Appendix

(5). Small Intestine

(6). Anus

(7). Descending Colon

(8). Sigmoid Colon

(9). Rectum

Spleen

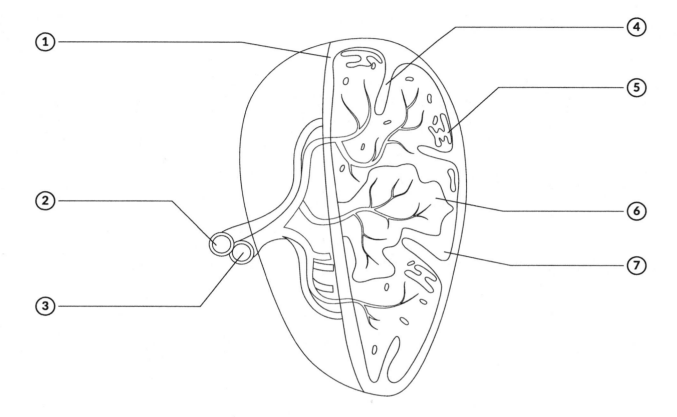

- - Answer - -

(1). Capsule

(2). Artery

(3). Vein

(4). Trabecula

(5). Vascular Sinusoid

(6). White Pulp

(7). Red Pulp

Gallbladder

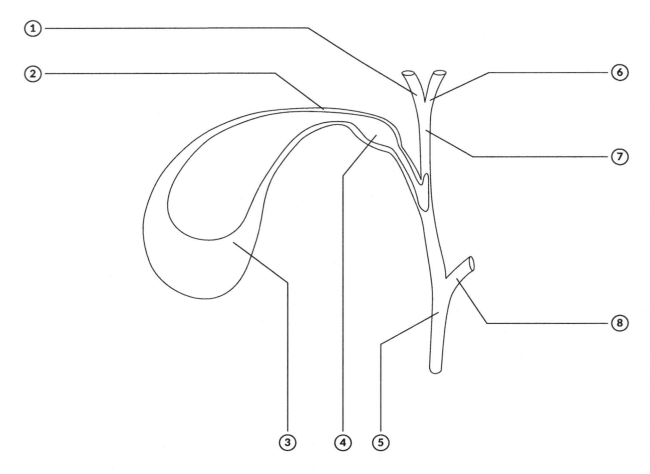

- - Answer - -

(1). Right Hepatic Duct   (5). Common Bile Duct

(2). Gallbladder Neck   (6). Left Hepatic Duct

(3). Gallbladder Body   (7). Common Hepatic Duct

(4). Cystic Duct   (8). Pancreatic Duct

Bronchial Tree

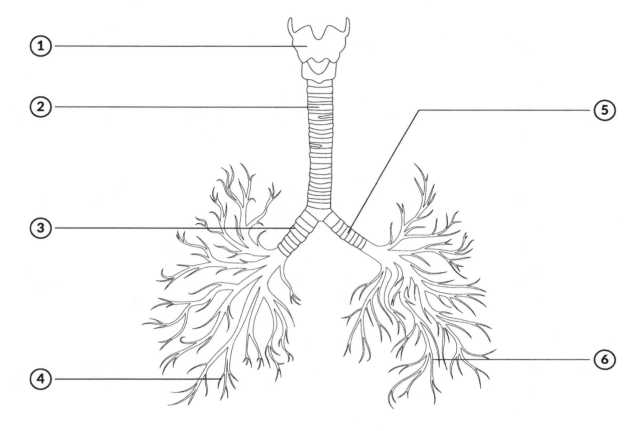

① ② ③ ④ ⑤ ⑥

- - Answer - -

(1).Larynx

(2).Trachea

(3).Right Main (Primary) Bronchus

(4).Bronchiole

(5).Left Main (Primary) Bronchus

(6).Tertiary Bronchus

Lymph Node

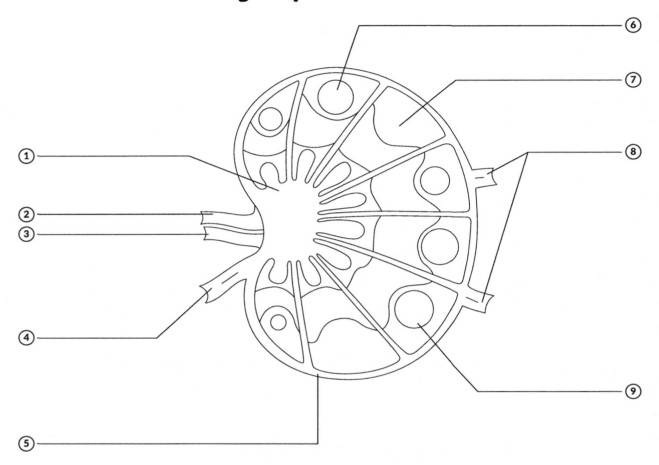

- - Answer - -

(1). Medullary Sinus

(2). Artery

(3). Vein

(4). Efferent Lymphatic Vessel

(5). Capsule

(6). Germinal Center

(7). Primary Lymphoid Follicle

(8). Afferent Lymphatic Vessel

(9). Secondary Lymphoid Follicle

Adrenal Gland

Adrenal Cortex :

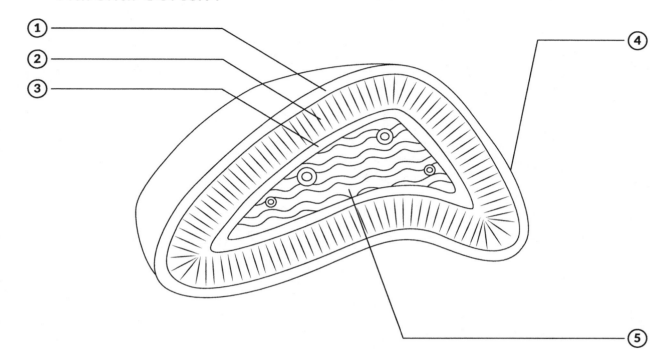

- - Answer - -

(1). Zona Glomerulosa

(2). Zona Fasciculata

(3). Zona Reticularis

(4). Capsule

(5). Medulla

Thyroid Gland

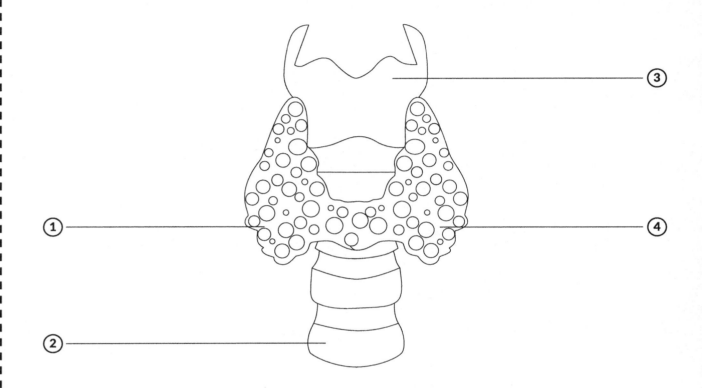

- - Answer - -

(1). Right Thyroid Gland

(2). Trachea

(3). Larynx

(4). Left Thyroid Gland

Interstitium

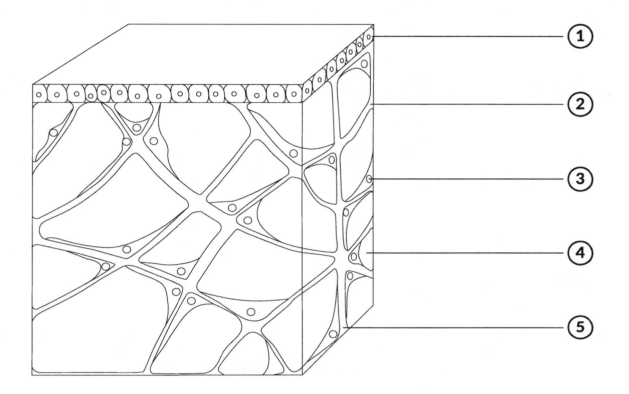

- - Answer - -

(1). Mucosa

(2). Collagen

(3). CD34 (Positive Form of Fibroblast)

(4). Fluid

(5). Elastin Fibers

Blood Vessels Structure

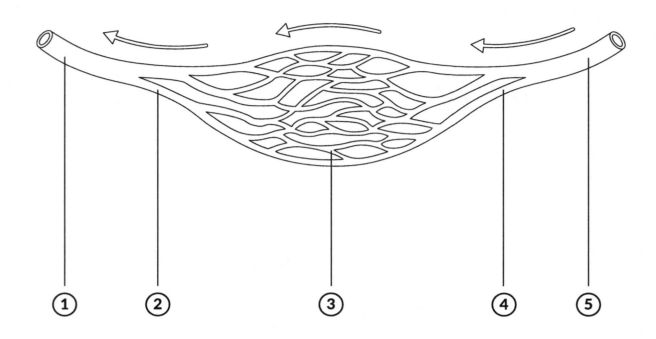

① ② ③ ④ ⑤

- - Answer - -

(1). Vein

(2). Venule

(3). Capillaries

(4). Arteriole

(5). Artery

Bone Marrow & Blood Cells

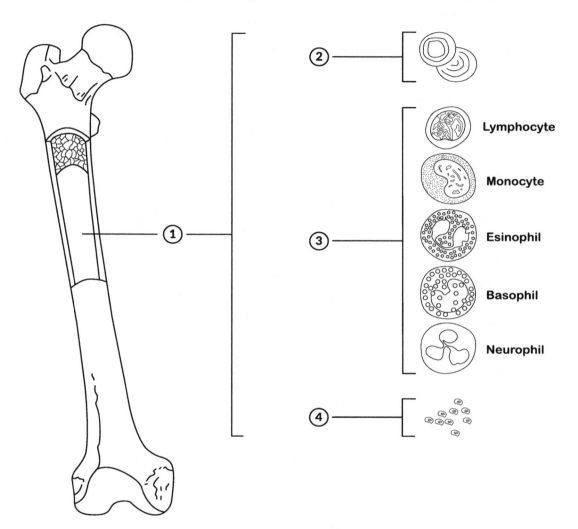

Lymphocyte

Monocyte

Esinophil

Basophil

Neurophil

- - Answer - -

(1). Marrow

(2). Red Blood Cells

(3). White Blood Cells

(4). Platelets

Artery

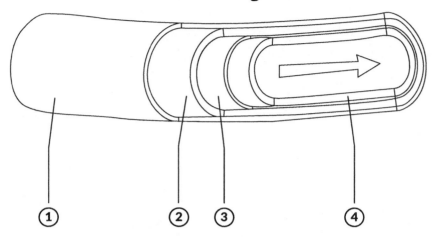

① ② ③ ④

Vein

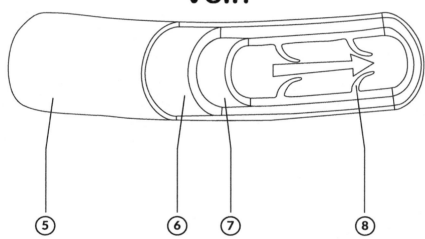

⑤ ⑥ ⑦ ⑧

- - Answer - -

Artery

(1). Outer Layer

(2). Smooth Muscle

(3). Elastic Layer

(4). Inner Layer

Vein

(5). Outer Layer

(6). Smooth Muscle

(7). Inner Layer

(8). Valve

Excretion

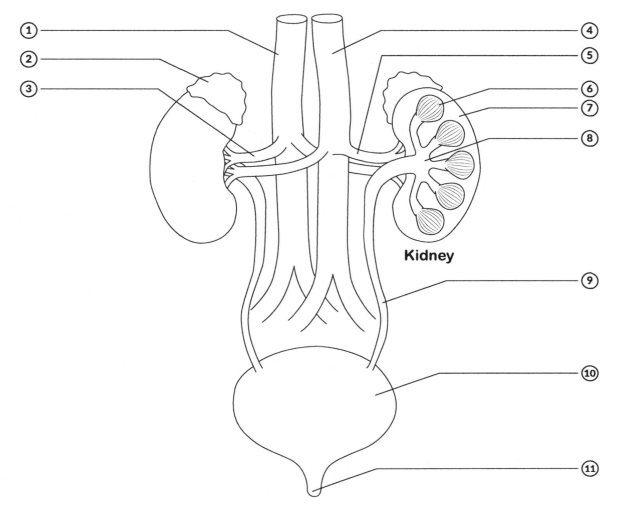

Kidney

- - Answer - -

(1). Inferior Vena Cava

(2). Adrenal Gland

(3). Renal Vein

(4). Aorta

(5). Renal Artery

(6). Medula

(7). Cortex

(8). Renal Pelvis

(9). Ureter

(10). Urinary Bladder

(11). Urethra

Male Pelvis

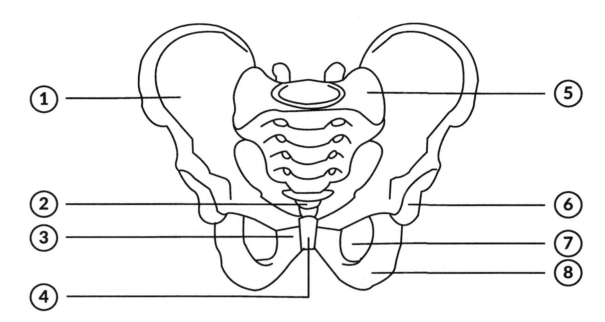

- - Answer - -

(1). Ilium

(2). Coccyx

(3). Pubis

(4). Symphysis Pubis

(5). Sacrum

(6). Acetabulum

(7). Obturator Foramen

(8). Ischium

Female Pelvis

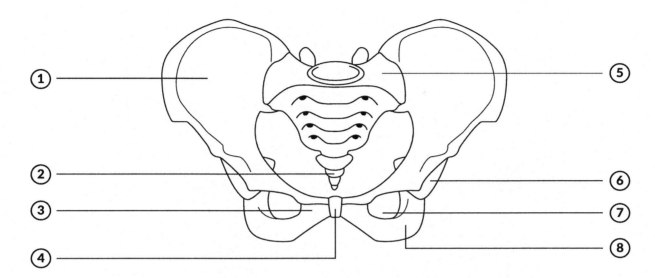

- - Answer - -

(1). Ilium

(2). Coccyx

(3). Pubis

(4). Symphysis Pubis

(5). Sacrum

(6). Acetabulum

(7). Obturator Foramen

(8). Ischium

Rib

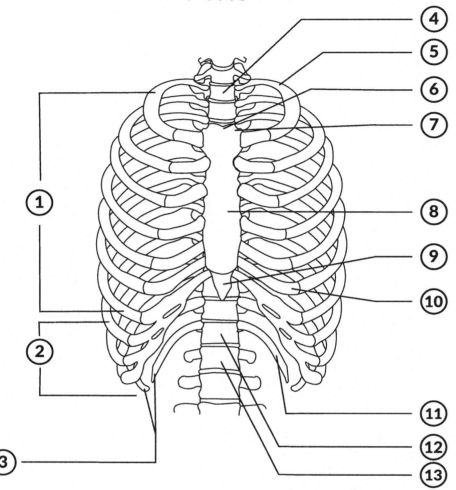

- - Answer - -

(1). True ribs (1-7)

(2). False ribs (8-12)

(3). Floating ribs (11 and 12)

(4). First thoracic vertebra

(5). First rib

(6). Jugular notch

(7). Clavicular notch

(8). Sternum

(9). Xiphoid process

(10). Costal cartilage

(11). Twelfth rib

(12). Twelfth thoracic vertebra

(13). First lumbar vertebra

Spine

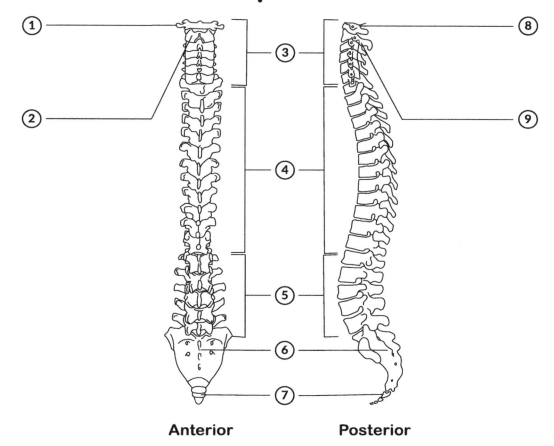

Anterior   Posterior

-- Answer --

(1). Atlas (first cervical vertebra)

(2). Axis (second cervical vertebra)

(3). Cervical vertebrae

(4). Thoracic vertebrae

(5). Lumbar vertebrae

(6). Sacrum

(7). Coccyx

(8). Atlas (first cervical vertebra)

(9). Axis (second cervical vertebra)

Anterior Shoulder

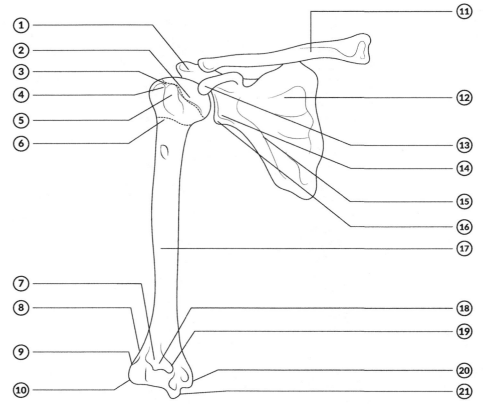

-- Answer --

(1). Acromion

(2). Humeral Head

(3). Anatomic Neck

(4). Greater Tubercle

(5). Lesser Tubercle

(6). Surgical Neck

(7). Radial Fossa

(8). Lateral Condyle

(9). Lateral Epicondyle

(10). Capitulum

(11). Clavicle

(12). Scapula

(13). Coracoid Process

(14). Infraglenoid Tubercle

(15). Subscapular Fossa

(16). Glenoid Cavity

(17). Humerus

(18). Coronoid Fossa

(19). Medial Condyle

(20). Medial Epicondyle

(21). Trochlea

Posterior Shoulder

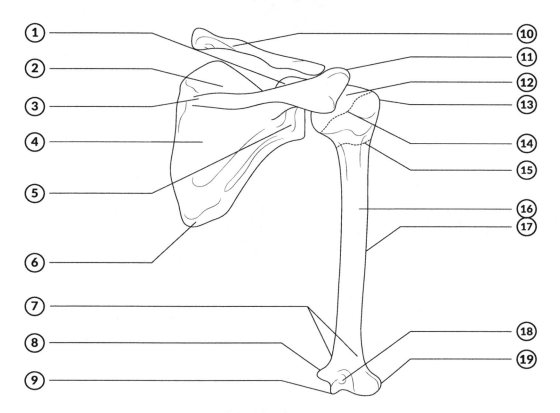

-- Answer --

(1). Coracoid Process

(2). Supraspinous Fossa

(3). Scapular Spine

(4). Scapula

(5). Scapular Neck

(6). Scapular Inferior Angle

(7). Supracondylar Ridge

(8). Medial Epicondyle

(9). Trochlea

(10). Clavicle

(11). Acromion Angle

(12). Humeral Head

(13). Greater Tubercle

(14). Anatomic Neck

(15). Surgical Neck

(16). Humerus

(17). Deltoid Tuberosity

(18). Olecranon Fossa

(19). Lateral Epicondyle

Nail

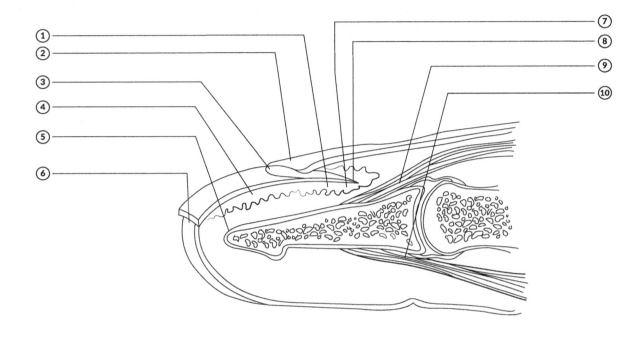

-- Answer --

(1). Germinai Matrix

(2). Eponychium

(3). Lunula

(4). Sterile Matrix

(5). Periosteum

(6). Hyponychium

(7). Ventral Floor

(8). Dorsal Root

(9). Extensor Tendon

(10). Flexor Tendon

Skull

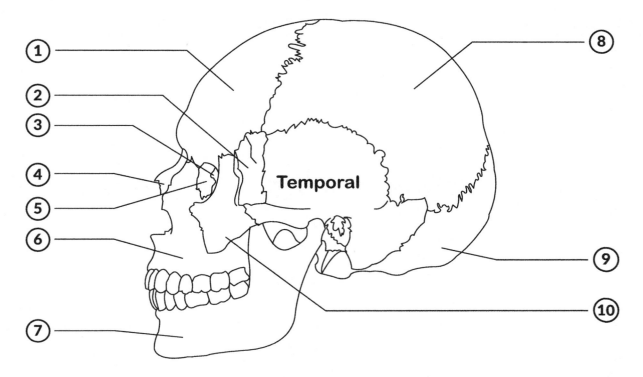

Temporal

- - Answer - -

(1). Frontal   (6). Maxilla

(2). Sphenoid   (7). Mandible

(3). Ethmoid   (8). Parietal

(4). Nasal   (9). Occipital

(5). Lacrimal   (10). Zygomatic

Anatomy (Larynx / Pharynx)

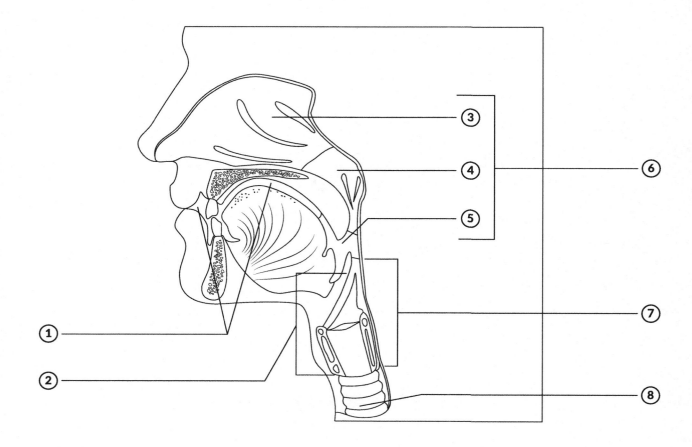

- - Answer - -

(1). Oral Cavity

(2). Larynx

(3). Nasal Cavity

(4). Nasopharynx

(5). Oropharynx

(6). Pharynx

(7). Hypopharynx

(8). Trachea

The Salivary Glands and The Blood Vessels of The Neck and Face.

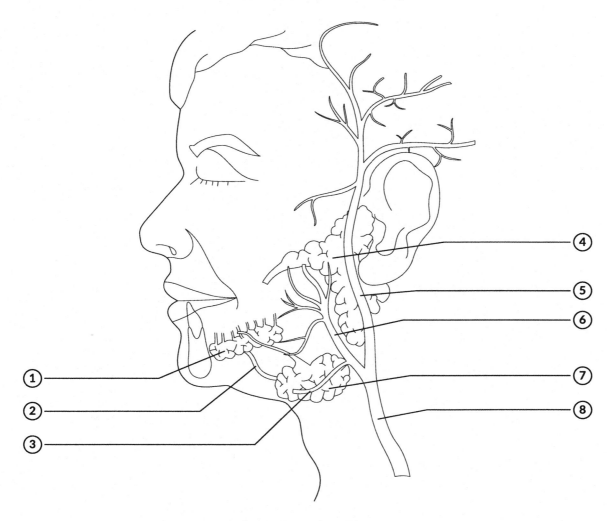

- - Answers - -

(1). Sublingual Gland

(2). Sublingual Artery

(3). Lingual Artery

(4). Parotid Gland

(5). Internal Carotid Artery

(6). External Carotid Artery

(7). Submandibular Gland

(8). Common Carotid Artery

Joints

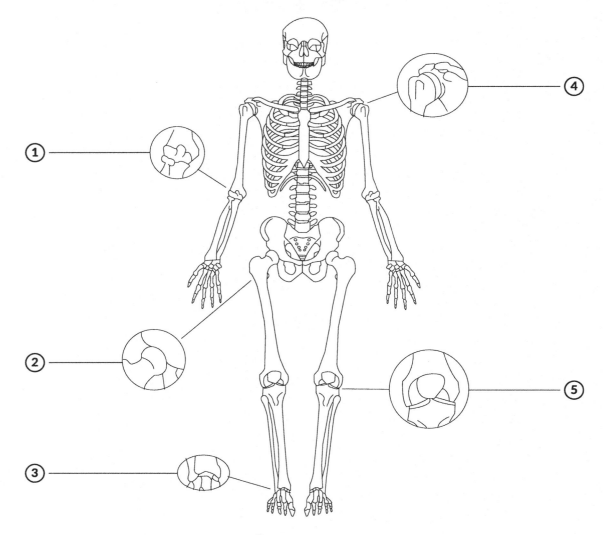

- - Answer - -

(1). Elbow Joint

(2). Hip Joint

(3). Ankle Joint

(4). Shoulder Joint

(5). Knee Joint

ELBOW JOINT

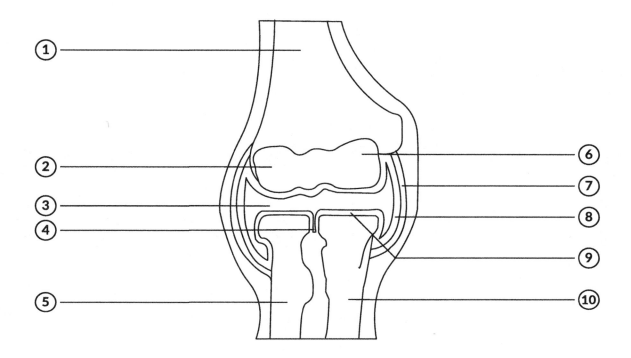

- - Answer - -

(1). Humerus

(2). Capitulum

(3). Synovia

(4). Proximal Radioulnar Joint

(5). Radius

(6). Trochlea

(7). Capsular Ligament

(8). Synovial Membrane

(9). Articular Cartilage

(10). Ulna

HIP JOINT

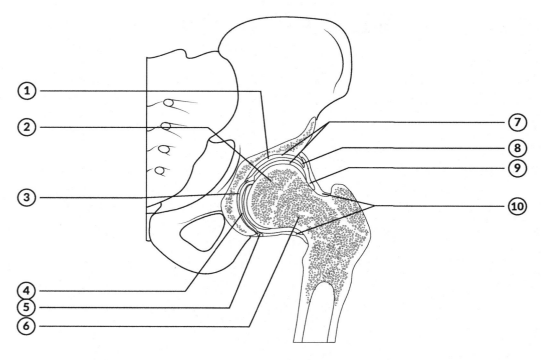

- - Answer - -

(1). Acetabulum

(2). Femoral Head

(3). Acetabular Fossa

(4). Ligament of The Head of The Femur

(5). Transverse Acetabular Ligament

(6). Femoral Neck

(7). Cartilage

(8). Acetabular Labrum

(9). Synovial Cavity

(10). Articular Capsule

ANKLE JOINT

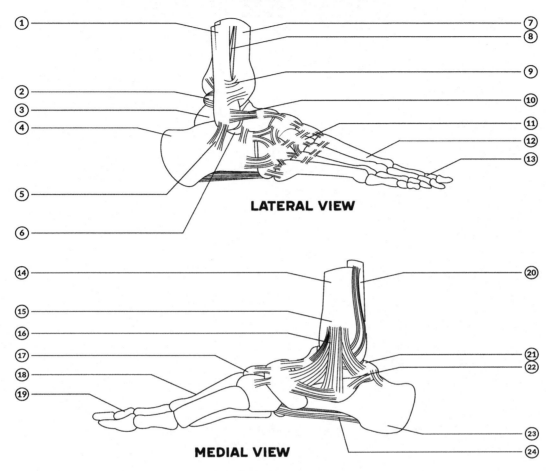

LATERAL VIEW

MEDIAL VIEW

- - Answer - -

(1). Fibula

(2). Posterior Inferior Tibiofibular Ligament

(3). Talus

(4). Calcaneus

(5). Calcaneofibular Ligament

(6). Subtalar Joint

(7). Tibia

(8). Interosseous Membrane

(9). Anterior Inferior Tibiofibular Ligament

(10). Anterior Talofibular Ligament

(11). Tarsals

(12). Metatarsals

(13). Phalanges

(14). Tibia

(15). Medial Malleolus

(16). Deltoid Ligament

(17). Tarsals

(18). Metatarsals

(19). Phalanges

(20). Fibula

(21). Talus

(22). Subtalar Joint

(23). Calcaneus

(24). Plantar Fascia

SHOULDER JOINT

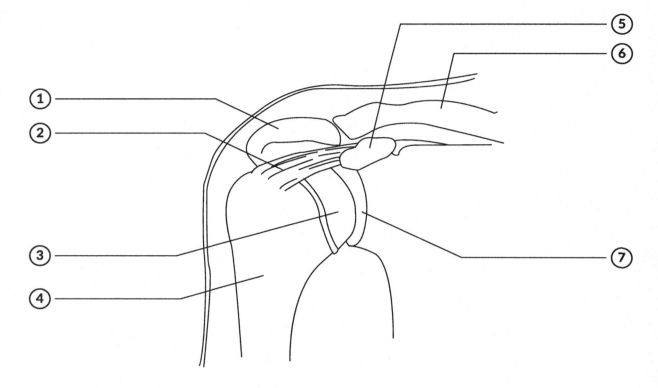

- - Answer - -

(1). Acromion

(2). Rotator Cuff

(3). Head of Humerus

(4). Humerus

(5). Coracoid Process

(6). Clavicle

(7). Glenoid

KNEE JOINT

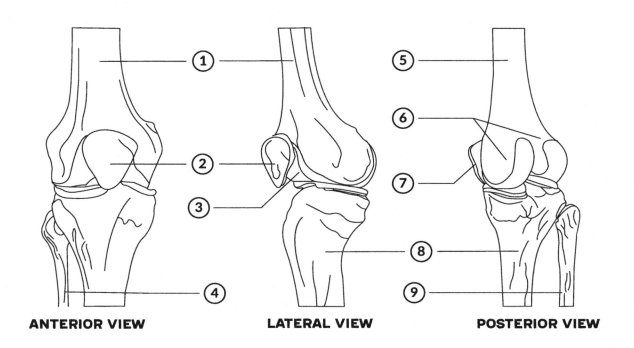

ANTERIOR VIEW   LATERAL VIEW   POSTERIOR VIEW

- - Answer - -

(1). Femur

(2). Patella

(3). Patellar Groove

(4). Fibula

(5). Femur

(6). Femoral Condyles

(7). Patella

(8). Tibia

(9). Fibula

Human Body Tissue Types

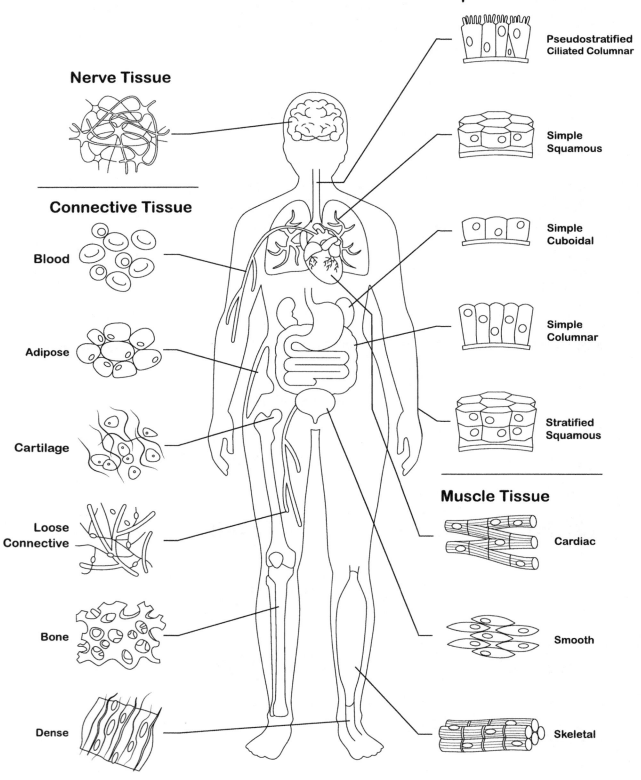

Epithelial Tissue

Pseudostratified Ciliated Columnar

Simple Squamous

Simple Cuboidal

Simple Columnar

Stratified Squamous

Nerve Tissue

Connective Tissue

Blood

Adipose

Cartilage

Loose Connective

Bone

Dense

Muscle Tissue

Cardiac

Smooth

Skeletal

Types of Connective Tissue

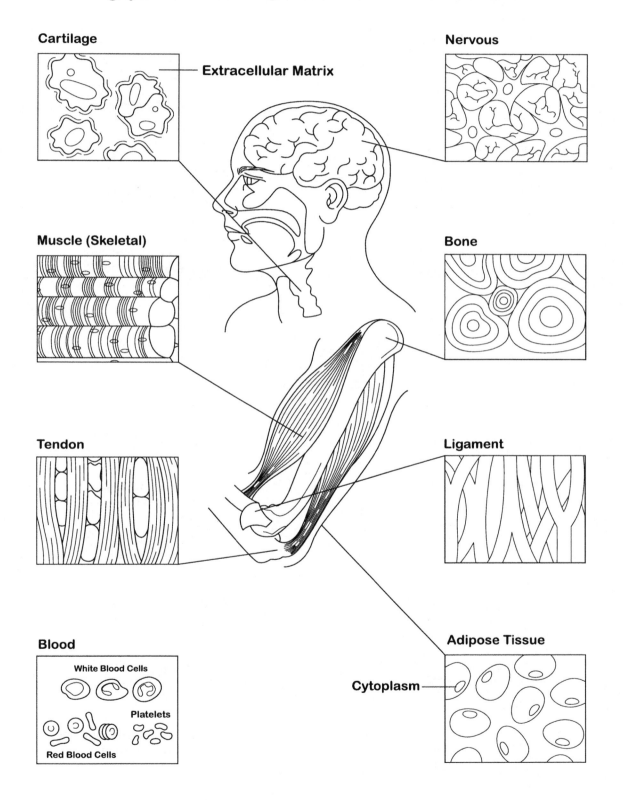

Cartilage

Extracellular Matrix

Nervous

Muscle (Skeletal)

Bone

Tendon

Ligament

Blood

White Blood Cells

Platelets

Red Blood Cells

Adipose Tissue

Cytoplasm

Types of Epithelial Tissue

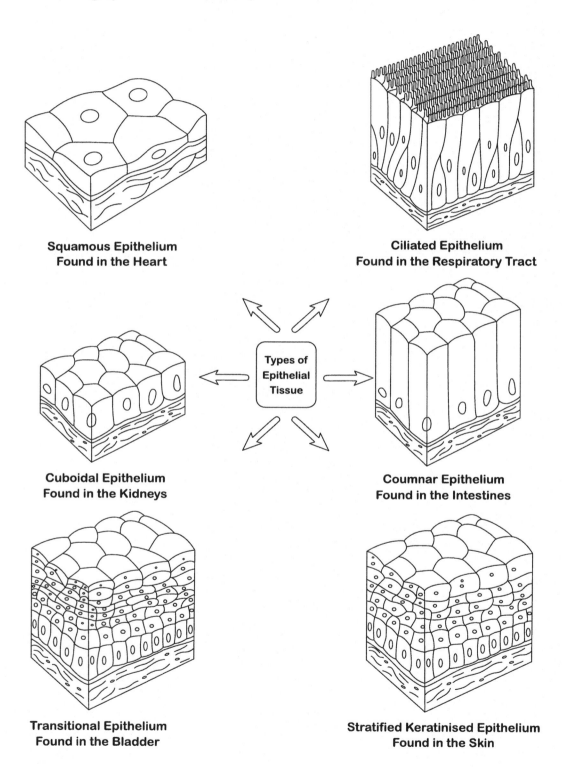

Squamous Epithelium
Found in the Heart

Ciliated Epithelium
Found in the Respiratory Tract

Types of
Epithelial
Tissue

Cuboidal Epithelium
Found in the Kidneys

Coumnar Epithelium
Found in the Intestines

Transitional Epithelium
Found in the Bladder

Stratified Keratinised Epithelium
Found in the Skin

Muscle Tissue

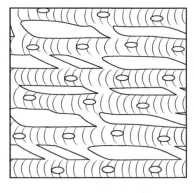

Cardiac Muscle

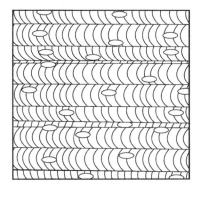

Skeletal Muscle

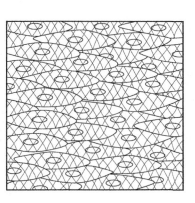

Smooth Muscle

Human Cells

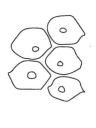

Skin Cells

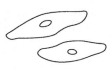

Red Blood Cells

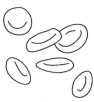

Smooth Muscle Cells

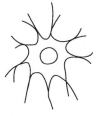

Bone

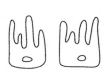

Epithelial Cells

Dendritic Cells

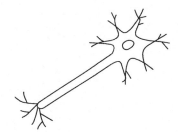

Nerve Cell

Stem Cell

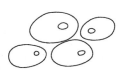

Fat Cells

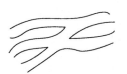

Heart Cell

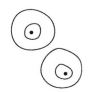

Ovum Cells

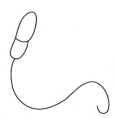

Sperm Cell

Neuron

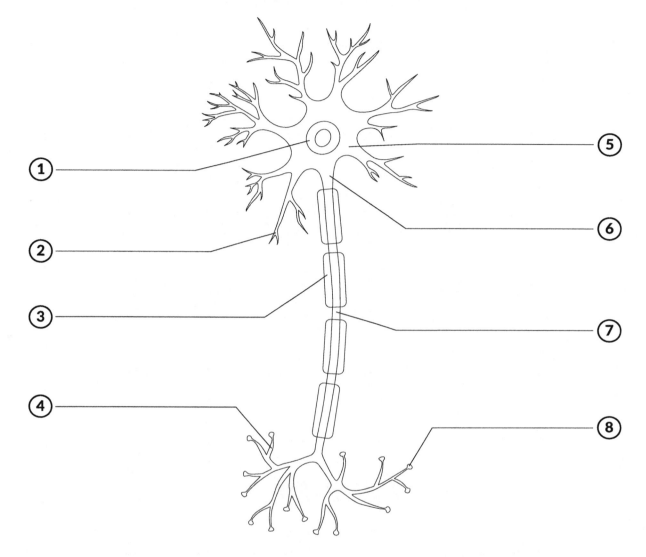

- - Answer - -

(1). Cell Body

(2). Dendrite

(3). Myelin Sheath

(4). Axon Terminal

(5). Nucleus

(6). Axon

(7). Node of Ranvier

(8). Synapse

Bones of The Face

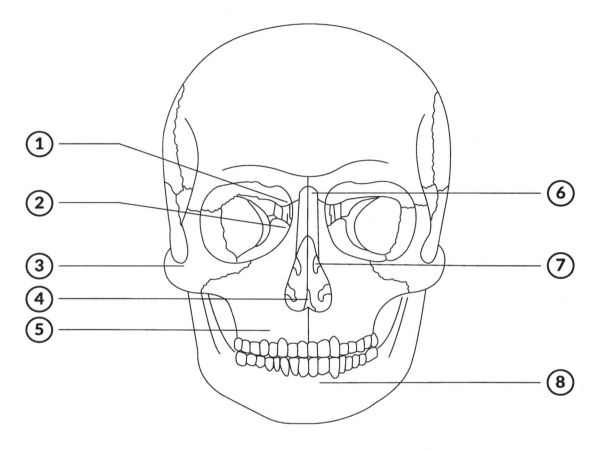

- - Answer - -

(1). Ethmoid

(2). Lacrimal

(3). Zygomatic

(4). Vomer

(5). Maxilla

(6). Nasal bone

(7). Turbinate

(8). Mandible

Bones of The Hand and Wrist

Posterior view

Anterior view

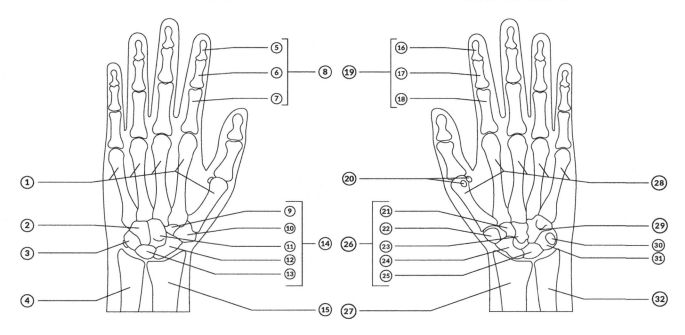

- - Answer - -

(1). Metacarpals

(2). Hamate

(3). Triquetrum

(4). Ulna

(5). Distal

(6). Middle

(7). Proximal

(8). Phalanges

(9). Trapezoid

(10). Trapezium

(11). Capitate

(12). Scaphoid

(13). Lunate

(14). Carpals

(15). Radius

(16). Distal

(17). Middle

(18). Proximal

(19). Phalanges

(20). Sesamoid bones

(21). Trapezoid

(22). Trapezium

(23). Capitate

(24). Scaphoid

(25). Lunate

(26). Carpals

(27). Radius

(28). Metacarpals

(29). Hamate

(30). Pisiform

(31). Triquetrum

(32). Ulna

Bones of The Hand

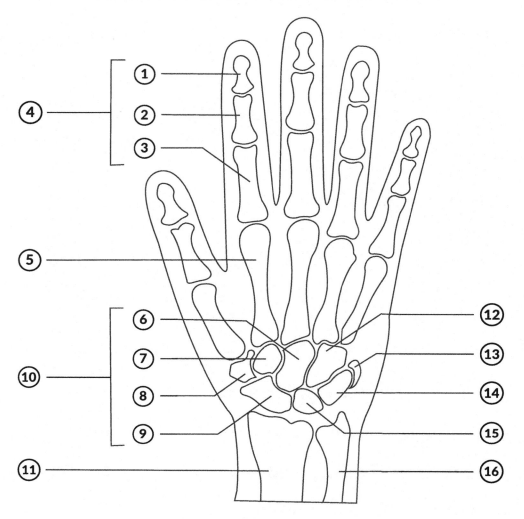

- - Answer - -

(1). Distal phalanx

(2). Middle phalanx

(3). Proximal phalanx

(4). Phalanges

(5). Metacarpal

(6). Capitate

(7). Trapezoid

(8). Trapezium

(9). Scaphoid

(10). Carpals

(11). Radius

(12). Hamate

(13). Pisiform

(14). Triquetral

(15). Lunate

(16). Ulna

Bones of The Arm

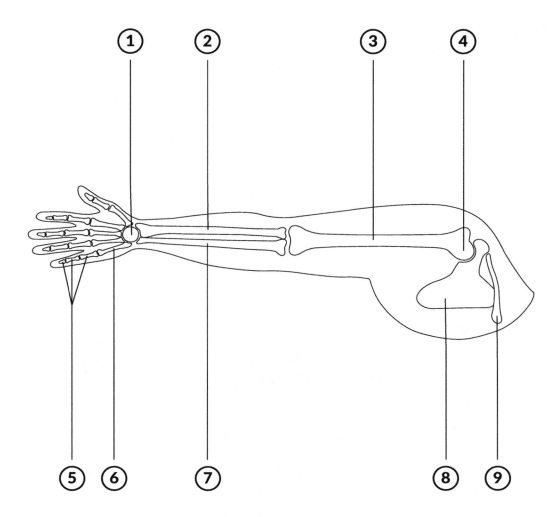

- - Answer - -

(1). Carpus

(2). Radius

(3). Humerus

(4). Rotator cuff

(5). Phalanges

(6). Metacarpus

(7). Ulna

(8). Scapula

(9). Clavicle

Bones of The Upper Limb

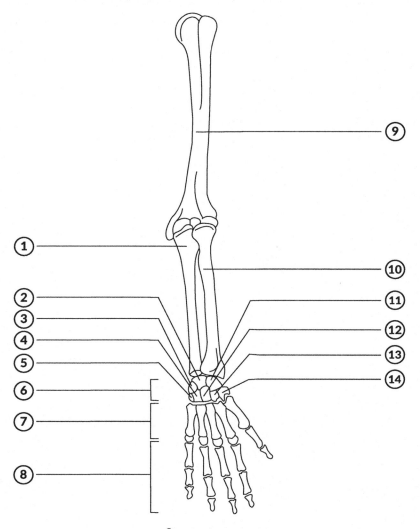

- - Answer - -

(1). Ulna

(2). Lunate

(3). Triquetral

(4). Hamate

(5). Pisiform

(6). Carpals

(7). Metacarpals

(8). Phalanges

(9). Humerus

(10). Radius

(11). Scaphoid

(12). Capitate

(13). Trapezoid

(14). Trapezium

Bones of the Foot

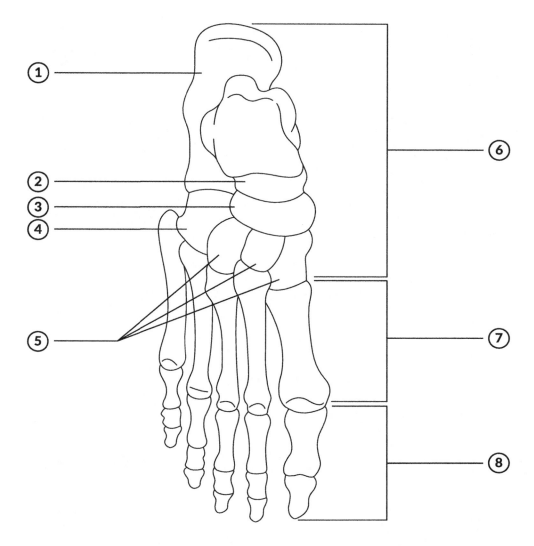

- - Answer - -

(1). Calcaneum (heel)

(2). Talus

(3). Navicular

(4). Cuboid

(5). Cuneiforms

(6). Tarsals

(7). Metatarsals

(8). Phalanges

Bones of The Foot

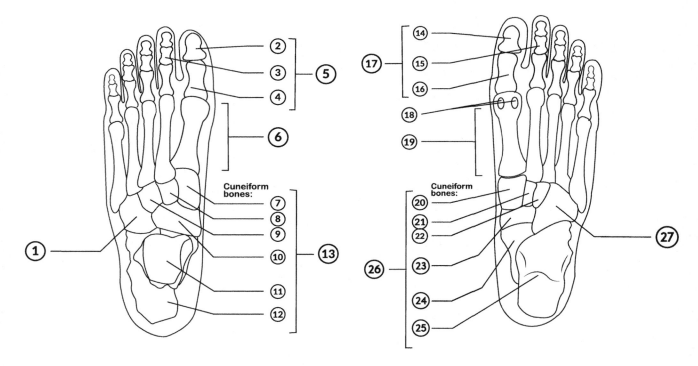

- - Answer - -

(1). Cuboid

(2). Distal

(3). Middle

(4). Proximal

(5). Phalanges

(6). Metatarsals

(7). Medial

(8). Intermediate

(9). Lateral

(10). Navicular

(11). Talus

(12). Calcaneus

(13). Tarsals

(14). Distal

(15). Middle

(16). Proximal

(17). Phalanges

(18). Sesamoid bones

(19). Metatarsals

(20). Medial

(21). Intermediate

(22). Lateral

(23). Navicular

(24). Talus

(25). Calcaneus

(26). Tarsals

(27). Cuboid

Foot Bones Front and Side

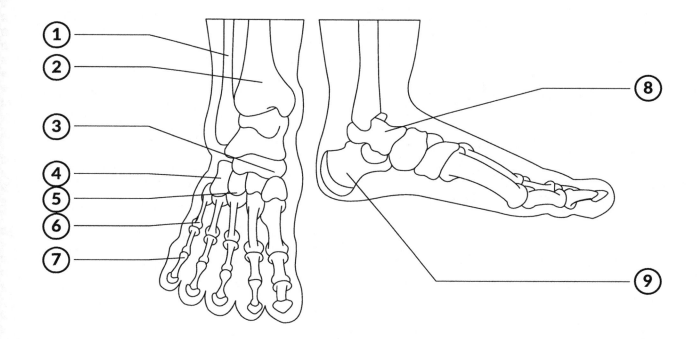

- - Answer - -

(1). Fibula

(2). Tibia

(3). Navicular bone

(4). Cuboid bone

(5). Cuneiform bone

(6). Metatarsal bone

(7). Phalange

(8). Talus

(9). Calcaneus

Knee Bones Front and Side

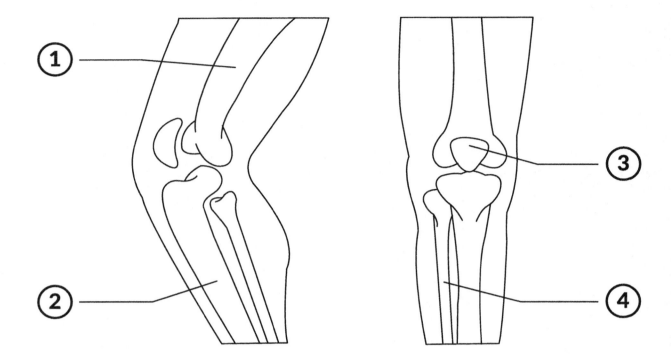

- - Answer - -

(1). Femur (thigh bone)

(2). Tibia (shin bone)

(3). Knee cap (patella)

(4). Fibula

Bones of The Lower Limb

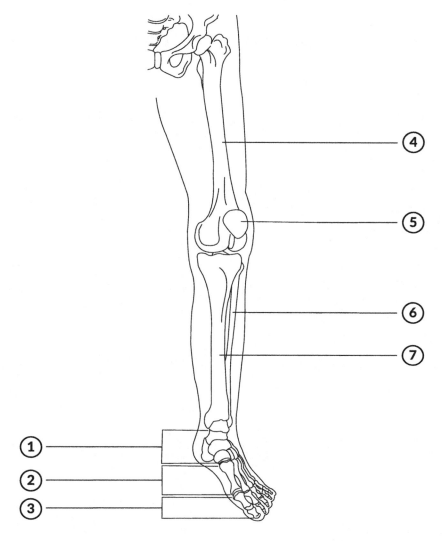

- - Answer - -

(1). Tarsals

(2). Metatarsals

(3). Phalanges

(4). Femur

(5). Patella

(6). Fibula

(7). Tibia

Muscles
Anterior View

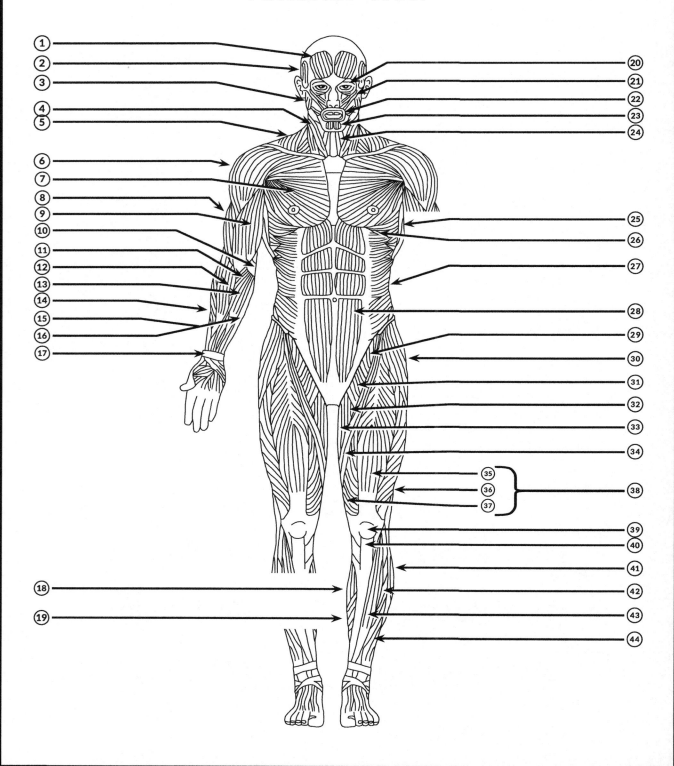

Muscles
Anterior View
- Answer -

(1). Frontalis

(2). Temporalis

(3). Masseter

(4). Sternocleidomastoid

(5). Trapezius

(6). Deltoid

(7). Pectoralis major

(8). Triceps brachii

(9). Biceps brachii

(10). Brachialis

(11). Pronator teres

(12). Brachioradialis

(13). Flexor carpi radialis

(14). Extensor carpi radialis longus

(15). Palmaris longus

(16). Flexor carpi ulnaris

(17). Flexor retinaculum

(18). Gastrocnemius

(19). Soleus

(20). Orbicularis oculi

(21). Zygomaticus

(22). Orbicularis oris

(23). Mentalis

(24). Sternohyoid

(25). Latissimus dorsi

(26). Serratus anterior

(27). External obliques

(28). Rectus abdominus

(29). Pectinius

(30). Tensor fasciae latae

(31). Adductor longus

(32). Adductor magnus

(33). Gracilis

(34). Sartorius

(35). Rectus femoris

(36). Vastus lateralis

(37). Vastus medialis

(38). Quadratus femoris

(39). Patella

(40). Patellar ligament

(41). Peroneus longus

(42). Extensor digitorum longus

(43). Tibialis anterior

(44). Peroneous tertius

Muscles

Posterior View

Muscles
Posterior View
- Answer -

(1). Flexor carpi ulnaris

(2). Extensor carpi ulnaris

(3). Extensor digitorum
Flexor retinaculum

(4). Gluteus medium

(5). Glutues maximus

(6). Adductor magnus

(7). Iliotibial tract

(8). Sartorius

(9). Semimembranosus

(10). Semitendinosus

(11). Biceps femoris

(12). Hamstrings

(13). Gastrocnemius

(14). Soleus

(15). Peroneus longus

(16). Achillestendon (Calcaneal tendon)

(17). Occipitalis

(18). Sternocleidomastoid

(19). Trapezius

(20). Deltoid

(21). Infraspinatus

(22). Teres major

(23). Rhomboid major

(24). Triceps brachii

(25). Latissimus dorsi

(26). Extensor carpi radialis longus

(27). Bracioradialis

(28). Flexor retinaculum

Muscles of the Anterior Neck, Shoulders, Chest and Thorax

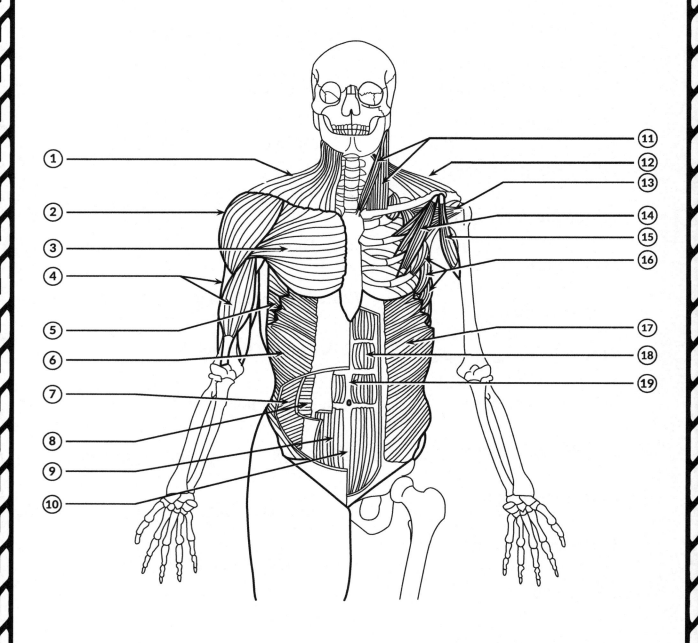

Muscles of the Anterior Neck, Shoulders, Chest and Thorax

- Answer -

(1). Platysma

(2). Deltoid

(3). Pectoralis major

(4). Biceps brachii

(5). Serratus anterior

(6). External oblique

(7). Internal oblique

(8). Transversus abdominus

(9). Rectus abdominus

(10). Linea alba

(11). Sternocleidomastoid

(12). Trapezius

(13). Subscapularis

(14). Pectoralis minor

(15). Coracobrachialis

(16). Serratus anterior

(17). External oblique

(18). Rectus abdominus

(19). Linea alba

Muscles of The Posterior Neck, Shoulders, and Thorax

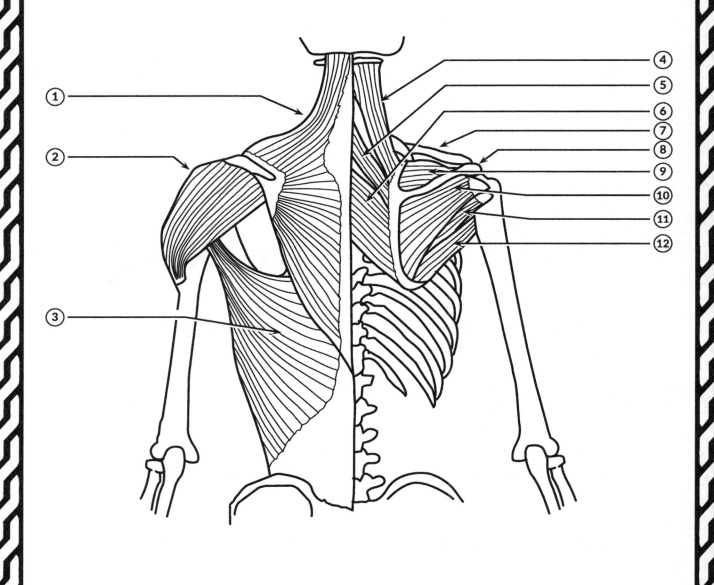

1
2
3
4
5
6
7
8
9
10
11
12

Muscles of The Posterior Neck, Shoulders, and Thorax

- Answer -

(1). Platysma

(2). Deltoid

(3). Latissimus dorsi

(4). Levator scapulae

(5). Rhomboid minor

(6). Rhomboid major

(7). Clavicle

(8). Scapular spine

(9). Supraspinatus

(10). Infraspinatus

(11). Teres minor

(12). Teres major

Muscles of The Face

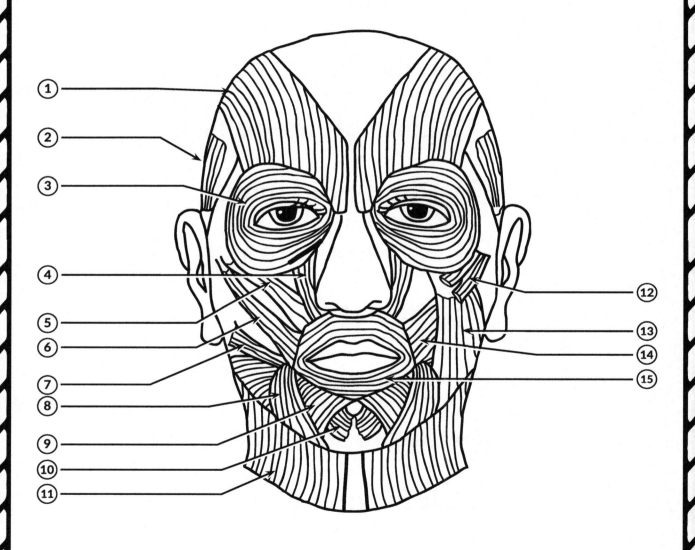

Muscles of The Face
- Answer -

(1). Frontalis

(2). Temporalis

(3). Orbicularis oculi

(4). Levator labii superioris

(5). Zygomaticus minor

(6). Zygomaticus major

(7). Risorius

(8). Depressor anguli oris (also called Triangularis)

(9). Depressor labii inferioris

(10). Mentalis

(11). Platysma

(12). Zygomaticus (cut)

(13). Masseter

(14). Buccinator

(15). Orbicularis oris

Muscles of the Anterior Arm and Forearm
(Most Superfical)

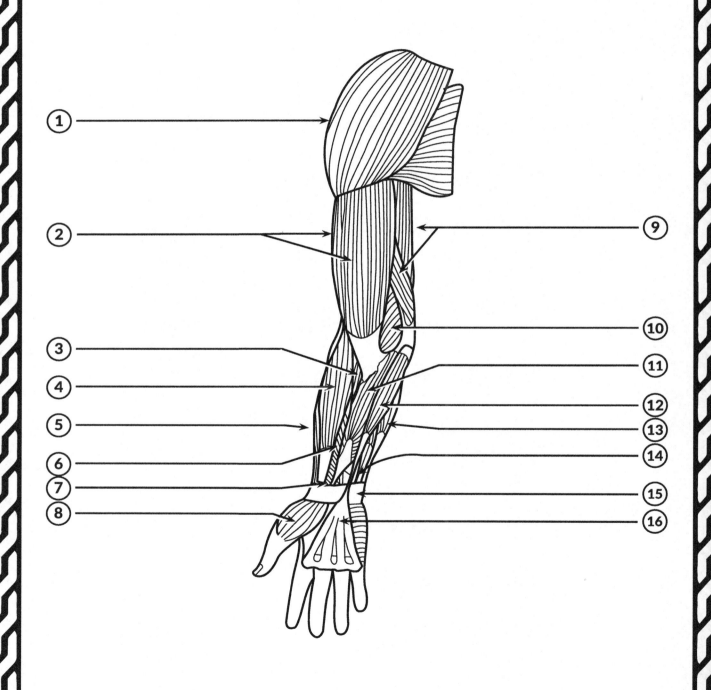

Muscles of the Anterior Arm and Forearm
(Most Superfical)
- Answer -

(1). Deltoid

(2). Biceps brachii

(3). Pronator teres

(4). Brachioradialis

(5). Extensor carpi radialis longus
(posterior - just visible here)

(6). Flexor pollicis longus

(7). Pronator quadratus

(8). Thenar muscles of the thumb

(9). Triceps brachii

(10). Brachialis

(11). Flexor carpi radialis

(12). Palmaris longus

(13). Flexor carpi ulnaris

(14). Flexor Digitorum superficialis
(deep to the above 3 muscles)

(15). Flexor retinaculum

(16). Palmar aponeurosis (fascia)

Muscles of the Posterior Arm and Forearm

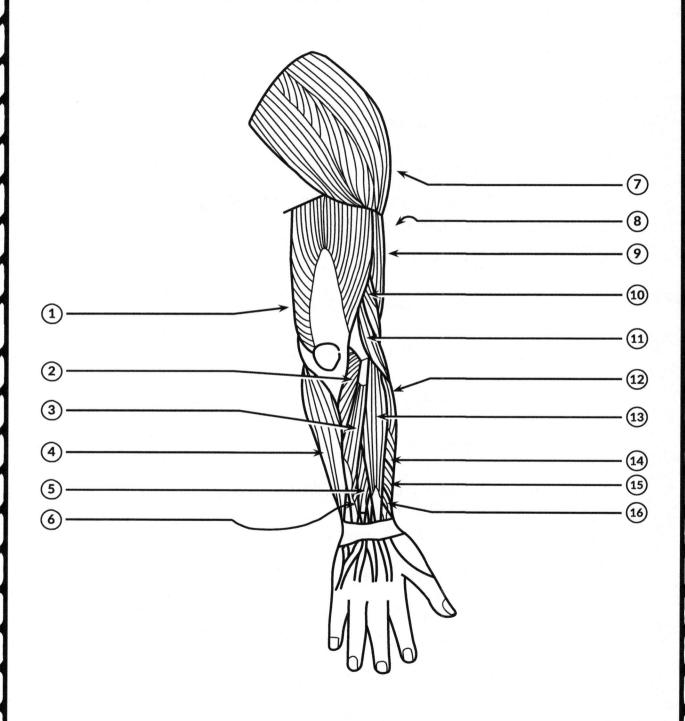

Muscles of the Posterior Arm and Forearm
- Answer -

(1). Triceps brachii

(2). Anconeus

(3). Extensor carpi ulnaris

(4). Flexor carpi ulnaris

(5). Extensor digiti minimi

(6). Extensor indicis (deep)

(7). Deltoid

(8). Biceps brachii (anterior)

(9). Brachialis

(10). Brachioradialis

(11). Extensor carpi radialis longus

(12). Extensor carpi radialis brevis

(13). Extensor digitorum

(14). Abductor pollicis longus

(15). Extensor pollicis brevis

(16). Extensor pollicis longus

Muscles of the Anterior Thigh
(and other important landmarks)

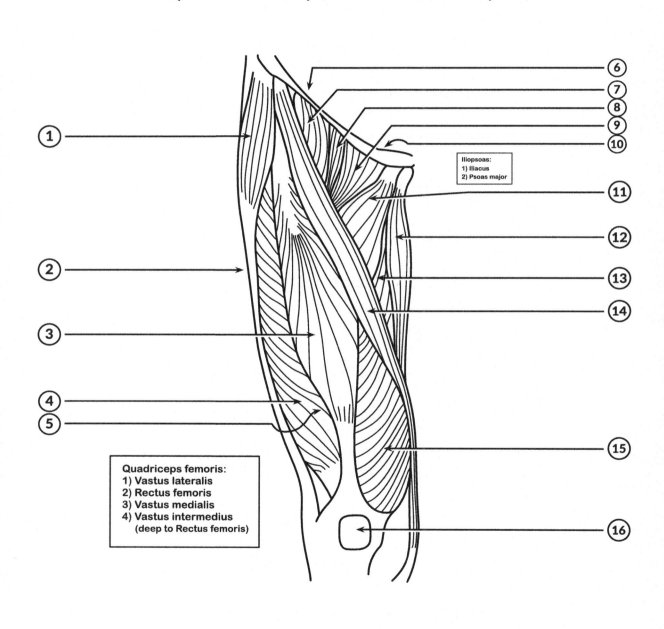

Iliopsoas:
1) Iliacus
2) Psoas major

Quadriceps femoris:
1) Vastus lateralis
2) Rectus femoris
3) Vastus medialis
4) Vastus intermedius
   (deep to Rectus femoris)

Muscles of the Anterior Thigh
(and other important landmarks)
- Answer -

(1). Tensor fasciae lata

(2). (Iliotibial tract)

(3). Rectus femoris

(4). Vastus lateralis

(5). Vastus intermedius
(deep to rectus femoris)

(6). (Inguinal ligament)

(7). Iliacus

(8). Psoas major

(9). Pectineus

(10). Adductor brevis
(deep beneath pectineus)

(11). Adductor longus

(12). Gracilus

(13). Adductor magnus

(14). Sartorius

(15). Vastus medialis

(16). (Patella)

Muscles of the Posterior Thigh
(and other important landmarks)

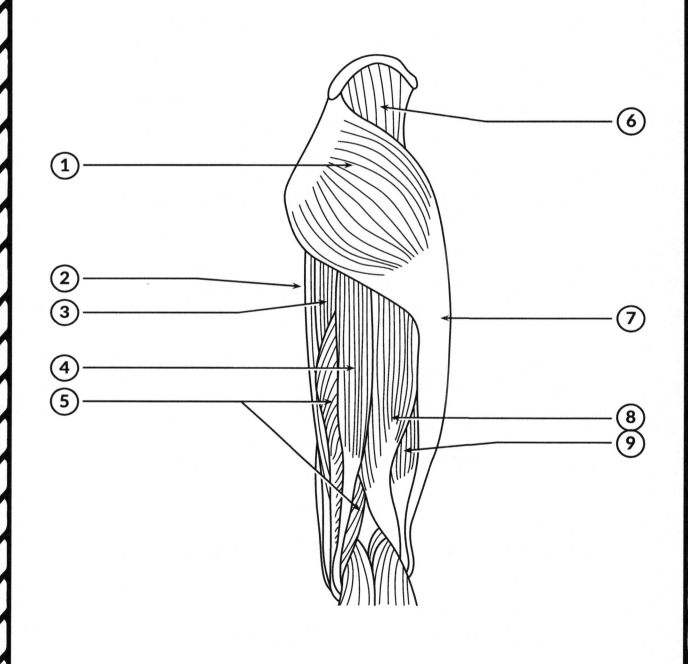

Muscles of the Posterior Thigh
(and other important landmarks)
- Answer -

(1). Gluteus maximus

(2). Gracilis

(3). Adductor magnus

(4). Semitendinosus

(5). Semimembranosus

(6). Gluteus medius

(7). (Iliotibial tract)

(8). Biceps femoris: Long head

(9). Short head

Muscles of the Leg (Calf) and Foot
(and other important landmarks)

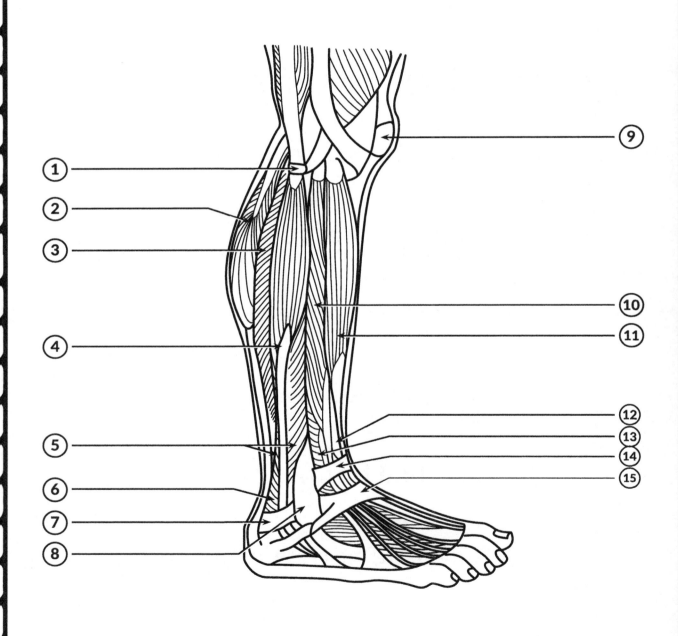

Muscles of the Leg (Calf) and Foot
(and other important landmarks)
- Answer -

(1). Head of the fibula

(2). Gastrocnemius

(3). Soleus

(4). Peroneus longus

(5). Peroneus brevis

(6). Flexor hallicus longus

(7). Peroneal retinaculum

(8). Lateral malleolus ("ankle bone")

(9). Patella

(10). Extensor digitorum longus

(11). Tibialis anterior

(12). Tensor hallicus longus

(13). Peroneus tertius

(14). Superior extensor retinaculum

(15). Inferior extensor retinaculum

Muscles of The Abdomen

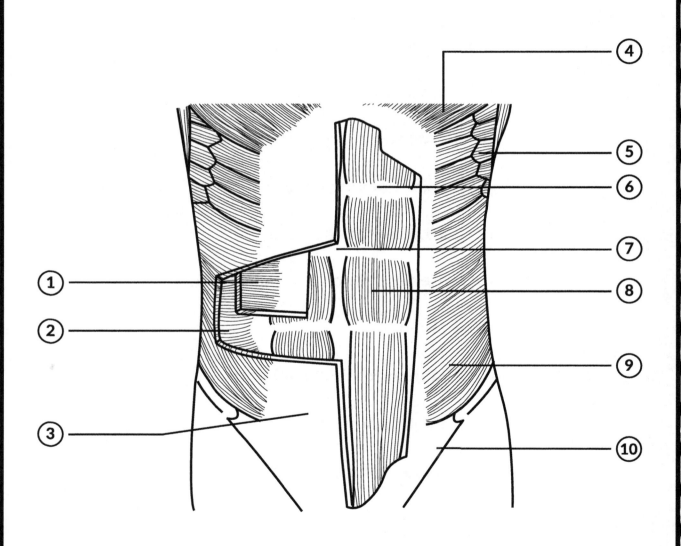

Muscles of The Abdomen
- Answer -

(1). Transversus abdominis

(2). Internal oblique

(3). Aponeurosis

(4). Pectoralis major

(5). Serratus anterior

(6). Tendinous intersection

(7). Linea alba

(8). Rectus abdominis

(9). External oblique

(10). Inguinal ligament

Muscle Types

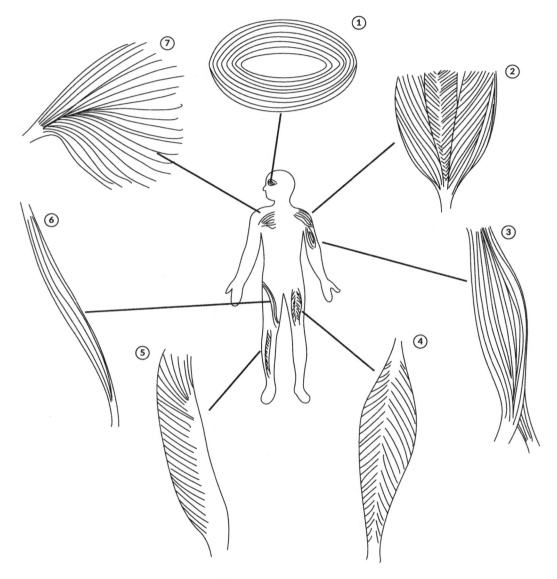

- Answer -

(1). Circular

(2). Multipennate

(3). Fusiform

(4). Bipennate

(5). Unipennate

(6). Parallel

(7). Convergent

Printed in Great Britain
by Amazon

41586604R00057